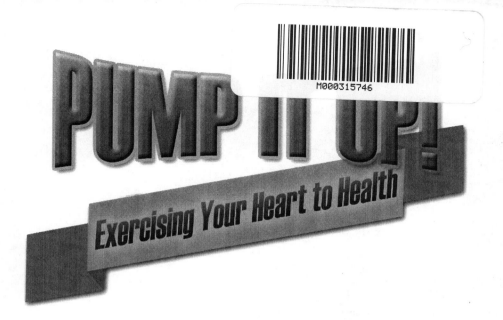

PUMP IT UP!
Exercising Your Heart to Health

Joe Petreycik, RN
ACSM Certified Clinical Exercise
Specialist[SM]

FOREWORD

By

Stuart W. Zarich, M.D.

Chief, Cardiovascular Medicine, Bridgeport Hospital
Yale New Haven Health

TAKE EXERCISE TO HEART, LLC
Stratford, Connecticut

DISCLAIMER:
Important note: Before beginning this or any exercise or diet program, it is important for you to see your internist or cardiologist for a routine physical to ensure your overall safety and fitness to start a workout regimen or a new diet plan.

Published by:
Take Exercise to Heart, LLC
7365 Main Street #323
Stratford, CT 06614 USA
www.exercisetoheart.com
e-mail: publisher@exercisetoheart.com

Print version
ISBN: 978-0-9894080-0-4 (trade paperback)
ISBN: 978-0-9894080-6-6 (hardcover)

E-book versions
ISBN: 978-0-9894080-1-1 (ebook)
ISBN: 978-0-9894080-2-8 (kindle)
ISBN: 978-0-9894080-3-5 (ePub)
ISBN: 978-0-9894080-4-2 (PDF merchant)

LCCN: 2013908981

Contents

Foreword

By

Stuart W. Zarich, M.D., FACC, FAHA, FASE
Chief, Cardiovascular Medicine
Bridgeport Hospital
Yale New Haven Health

Pump It Up! is an outstanding new book, written by Joseph Petreycik, who is not only a registered nurse, but a clinical exercise specialist. Joe relies on his experience as a registered nurse in cardiac rehabilitation and as an avid exercise enthusiast to present a comprehensive plan for enhancing cardiovascular health along the entire continuum of cardiovascular disease. Whether you are focusing on primary prevention, secondary prevention from a recent heart attack, or you are undergoing rehabilitation, this book contains something for everyone.

The book first gives you a better understanding of just what heart disease is and how a normal heart functions, and then goes into the importance of exercise and cardiac risk factor modification. *Pump It Up!* is filled with clinical vignettes, which I am sure many people will be able to relate to. The book is really a call to educating patients about the entire spectrum of cardiovascular disease, including sections on understanding cardiac medications and helping patients to take control of modifying their cardiac risk factors. An in-depth discussion of diet and nutrition is also included, which is typically lacking in a book stressing exercise.

This book helps to empower patients and to make them accountable for their health through education to understanding cardiac risk factors, symptomatology, how cardiac disease is diagnosed, and even what normal coronary anatomy looks like. However, the real strength of the book relies on its in-depth discussion of resistance training, which is often overlooked as compared to aerobic training. Most lay people understand the benefits of aerobic exercise to improve heart health, but know little regarding the benefits of resistance training.

Pump It Up! also goes into detail regarding the appropriate frequency, duration and intensity of exercise. I think what is little appreciated is how resistance training can be accomplished safely at home without a fancy gym or expensive equipment. More and more data are now available on the long-term benefits of resistance training, in addition to aerobic exercise, yet too few patients with cardiovascular disease maintain any resistance training. This book also blends the need to remain flexible and discusses the role of stretching and prevention of injuries while training.

In summary, the strength of *Pump It Up!* is to make an "educated consumer or best customer" in the medical profession. People need to understand what cardiovascular disease is, what are its particular risk factors, and how they can tackle these risks through healthy lifestyle modifications, including diet, stress reduction, exercise, and weight maintenance.

Joe is to be commended on his comprehensive approach to educating patients regarding disease processes, evaluation and treatments, and what they can do themselves as far as exercise, diet and nutrition are concerned to reduce their risk of heart disease.

Introduction

D o any of the following situations apply to you?

- You're overweight and you promise yourself that you'll add exercise to your schedule but you haven't gotten around to it.
- You've had a heart "incident" and your doctor advises you to start exercising, but where do you begin?
- You're recovering from a heart attack and you've been advised to lose weight and add exercise to your daily regimen.
- You are in good shape and you exercise regularly, but your exercises are not specifically designed to help keep your heart healthy, and you'd like to change that.

It is to address these and related concerns that I have spent the last six years researching and writing this book, based on my eight years of experience as a registered nurse specializing in clinical exercise. (For more information on my credentials and background, please see "About the Author" in the back of this book).

The information in this book, including the real-life examples that you will find in it, is based on my professional experiences. I know that this program works because it has worked for the hundreds of clients I have worked with over these eight years; it also has personally worked for me. Not only am I in excellent shape in terms of my stamina and muscle strength, but I have been able to drop 60 pounds and over 15% body fat by following the nutritional and exercise guidelines that you will learn in this book.

By reading *Pump it Up!* you will have at your fingertips a comprehensive plan for enhancing your health, along with strategies you can use for a longer and healthier life through exercise and diet. Congratulations on taking the first step in this exciting journey!

A key purpose of this book is to assist those who have cardiovascular disease (CVD), as well as other serious heart-related illnesses, who are beginning or resuming an exercise program. CVD includes coronary heart disease (CHD), congestive heart failure (CHF), angina pectoris (AP), myocardial infarction (MI) and stroke.[1] However, any illness caused by a problem with the heart and major blood vessels (arteries and veins), can be recognized as CVD.

As you probably know, heart disease remains the No.1 killer in the United States. (It is a major cause of a shorter life span internationally as well). Twelve percent (12%) of adults ages 18 and older have been told they have heart disease. Twenty-five percent (25%) have been told on two or more visits to their physician that they have high blood pressure. Three percent (3%) have been told they have experienced a stroke.[2]

Although evidence supports the benefits of a cardiac rehabilitation program consisting of monitored exercise, stress reduction and nutritional education classes for reducing the morbidity and mortality associated with CVD, overall attendance at such programs is poor.[1,3]

A Mayo Clinic study found cardiac rehab after an MI underused, particularly among females and the elderly. Females were 55% less likely than males to participate in cardiac rehab, and only 32% of the males and females 70 years of age or older participated in such programs compared to 66% of those in the 60-69-year age groups. The best participation rates, 81%, were among those up to 60 years of age.[4]

Important caveat: I want to make it very clear, however, that this book is *not* intended to replace a cardiac rehab program. Anyone who is eligible for such a program should make every effort to attend it. Such programs employ nurses and exercise physiologists working closely with physicians and their patients to devise the safest and most effective exercise plan to lower the risk of a future cardiac event. The self-confidence and support from these health care professionals usually justifies the time that is invested.

But for those who are unable to attend such a program due to a lack of medical insurance coverage, high deductibles or sky-rocketing co-pays, or for those who are attending a program but who would still like to learn more about creating and following a heart-healthy exercise and diet program that they can follow on their own, the principles you will learn in this book will provide you with that information.

This book will also benefit those who have already been in a cardiac rehab program, where you've worked with a nurse and exercise physiologist. If you have already successfully completed such a program, this book can be used as a welcome reference, reminding you of the principles that you learned in your program, as you now continue to carry on a program of your own.

For those new to exercise, *upon getting clearance from your doctor*, in addition to reading this book on your own, you may want to consider working with a clinical exercise physiologist who can provide you with additional support and guidance. If a clinical exercise physiologist has not been assigned to you, you will find suggestions in this book about how to find such a professional through your cardiologist, your local hospital or medical center, or through a related national association.

This book can also be a benefit to those without CVD, but who may have other risk factors for developing heart disease, such as obesity, type I or II diabetes mellitus, hypertension, high cholesterol, smoking, physical inactivity, family history, or advanced age, by showing you various workouts that can be performed in your local gym or even in the comfort of your own home.

As you read on, you will find a great deal of attention is devoted to strength training. Not only is this due to the importance of learning and implementing proper technique, but to reap the heart-strengthening benefits and maintain physical independence as we age. Research is showing how strength training can prevent a significant loss of strength as we age, reducing our risk of frailty thus enhancing our quality of life.[5]

You will also find in this book a nutritional guide to remind you of heart-healthy foods to include in your diet.

Finally, in this book you will be introduced to helpful stress-reduction techniques which can be incorporated into your daily life.

Part 1 of this book, "The Heart of the Matter," provides up-to-date medical information, including a discussion of heart anatomy, along with original illustrations to help you gain a better understanding of your heart and how it works. There is also a summary discussion of heart-related illnesses, risk factors and treatments. This part offers you the tools to better appreciate your body and your illness, and to ultimately help you understand the subsequent chapters of this book.

Part 2, "Exercise," delves into the all-important central fitness portion of the book. After reviewing the general benefits and barriers to exercise, you are provided with the tools to create a balanced program.

Part 3, "Special Considerations," begins with Chapter 12, "Understanding Your Medications and Their Implications for Your Exercise Routines," a discussion of medications that you might be taking and how they might impact your exercise routine.

Chapter 13, "Diet & Nutrition," is a review of the essentials of nutrition and decodes the many diets readily available to you to effectively create a heart-healthy, personalized diet.

The final chapter, Chapter 14, "Going Forward," shares another extensive informative case history; it also discusses additional concerns as you go forward with the plan that this book has started you on.

In the Appendix you will read a case history as well as sample workouts. Recommended Readings, Resources, an Index, and, finally, About the Author, which describes my background and credentials in greater length.

At various points throughout *Pump it Up!* you will read quotes from interviews I conducted with some of the cardiac rehab clients that I've worked with. One of the greatest benefits of a cardiac rehab program is that it can provide a strong support system and camaraderie among its participants. I hope you will find inspiration from their stories as you see that you are not alone in your quest to eat a more heart-friendly diet and as you *Pump it Up!: Exercising Your Heart to Health*.

To protect the identity of my exercise patients, pseudonyms are used; identifying details were also changed, if necessary, to protect their privacy. Other than those changes, or editing for length, the facts and words in their stories are as they were told to me. Although their identities are not shared, their contributions to this book are acknowledged with my thanks.

Part 1

The Heart of the Matter

Chapter 1

Saved by a heart Attack – A Father/Son Story

John is a successful business owner in business plan development and analysis, financial information marketing, and distribution content publishing. He was 52 years old and recovering from a heart attack when he and I first started working together. Despite his busy lifestyle working a full-time job to provide for his family, John made a commitment to exercise in the cardiac rehab program.

What John was able to accomplish in several months of enrollment in the cardiac rehab exercise program is a true testament to his dedication. Here is his story[*]:

> I sat on the edge of the paper-covered bench in the exam room, watching as my doctor examined the graph from the electrocardiogram machine. Well-known for his rapid diagnoses, he glanced at the paper stream in his hands for only a second or so and then said to me with some surprise, "It looks like you've had a heart attack."
>
> A heart attack. It was the phrase that I had been fearing for many months. In February of that year, I had been running to catch a train to New York City, pushing my overweight, desk-jockey body far harder than I would usually push it. I made the train with no time to spare, gasping for breath inside the coach car as the train doors closed behind me. "Are you all right?" a few of the passengers asked. "I'm fine, I just have to catch my breath," I said, and after a few minutes I found a seat and rested on the way in to the city.
>
> But I was not all right. I knew it at the time, but never having had anything remotely like a major medical problem in my life before, and being only 52 years old at the time, I really wasn't thinking that it was really possible for me to have a heart attack. After all, I had been eating pretty healthily…hadn't I? And yes, in the push to get work done, I had let my exercise lag for many years and put on a lot of weight, but I was still young. I could handle this. I sat through a lunch with a business

---

[*] I interviewed John, a pseudonym for his real name, and transcribed that interview. It is reprinted here, with minimal editing, for the sake of accuracy and to conceal or change any potentially identifiable details, with John's permission. Any additions in brackets are for clarity.

prospect, trying to focus on getting a contract with them for new work. The meeting went well. But I felt ... funny.

Weeks and months passed, and I continued to feel a little off, not in a way that I could put my finger on, but definitely feeling winded and ill-focused at times. But I was busy, and, after all, business had to come first if I was to take care of my family. During the summer months my 21-year-old son and I would go out sailing. But that summer I found it very difficult to raise the sails in the choppy waters of Long Island Sound, afraid that I was going to lose my balance in a way that I had not experienced before. But still, I did nothing.

Finally, in November, I got an exam for an insurance policy that required an electrocardiogram. The technician administering the test in our home wasn't there to read the results, only to collect the data. As I lay on our living room sofa while the machine read my heartbeat, I was saying to myself, "Please don't find a heart attack."

After seeing my doctor a couple of weeks later, he referred me to a heart specialist to confirm his diagnosis. In the specialist's office, I was put through tests on a treadmill with monitoring leads hanging off of my chest. A short while later, I was sitting in an exam room, hearing the words coming from the specialist's mouth, yet not quite absorbing it all. "Heart attack ... blockage ... procedure ... stents ... hospital ... as soon as possible." I put on my shirt and started to cry. I had tried so hard to do my best for my family, but instead of taking care of them, I had put them in danger. My wife nearly lost a husband and my son nearly lost a father. How could I have let them down like this? I felt very ashamed that I had not taken care of someone who was so important to them — me.

A few days later, I found myself at our local hospital, being wheeled into an operating room for the surgical procedure to insert my stents. The doctor explained how they would snake a probe up through an artery in my leg into my heart to insert the stents. I understood what was being done well enough, though the "twilight sleep" medications that they had given me made it difficult to understand exactly how long the procedure was taking.

I could see on the monitor in the operating room the image of my heart beating. Then, after some conversation between the doctor and the operating team, the picture on the monitor changed. I could see the squiggly outlines of my heart's arteries more clearly. The blockages in my arteries had been opened by the stents — I was seeing the blood flowing into my heart muscles again, feeding them with oxygen. Soon afterwards,

I was resting in my hospital room, watching the heart monitor beeping away and showing a blood pressure reading that I hadn't seen since my twenties and breathing deeply.

I realized right away that this was an amazing gift that I had received. It was like getting a second chance at life. One of my heart's arteries had had a 99.9% blockage and another had been 85% blocked. I was headed towards an untimely death. Now I had a heart that was getting fresh blood like it hadn't felt in years. Fortunately it turned out that my heart attack had not been too severe. My prognosis was good — if I followed directions. The next morning I was outside the hospital, waiting. for my wife to bring the car around.

As I stood in the cool, foggy morning air, I breathed in the fresh air deeply, knowing that every breath that I took, and every beat of my heart, was a blessing.

After I got home from the hospital, I ordered a Nintendo Wii™ game console and the Wii Fit™ software and equipment that worked with this unit. I had heard that the Wii Fit™ was a fun way to begin exercising and to sharpen your sense of balance. I bought it for my son as a Christmas present, hoping to get him interested in the exercise routines and active games that came with this machine. He wasn't too interested in the exercise software at first, but he was very interested in the sports and games that came with the Wii. Pretty soon we were playing active games together like we hadn't done since he was a small boy, except now that he was a young adult, we were playing much more actively and competitively. We began relating to one another in ways that we hadn't had a chance to try out in years past — I had been too busy with work and he had been too busy with college.

In addition to starting exercise, I also made some important changes in my diet. Both my wife's family and my family were big eaters in their own ways, each with their "bad for you" foods from their family traditions. My own habits for meals and snacking weren't any better, with too many sweets, starches, animal fat, and snacks.

Sugar, most animal fats and refined carbohydrates were out. Whole grains, nuts, soy products, fruits and vegetables were in. Portions got smaller. And I learned to say "no" to foods that weren't good for me with more conviction — and with more cooperation from family members.

I started to learn how to eat to live, rather than living to eat. I made important exceptions for holidays, birthdays and special celebrations, but for my first year after the surgery, I was very strict about following a very healthy diet. Very quickly I learned to like it. I really felt a lot better eating healthy foods.

A few weeks after Christmas, I started exercising at the cardio fitness center in the building where my heart specialist had his offices. The prescription from my heart specialist was to attend 36 sessions of cardio fitness training. I was eager to start this routine, though I wasn't so sure how well I would do at it. It felt funny strapping on the heart monitoring equipment and applying the leads to my chest. But the staff was very helpful, positive and supportive and they monitored everyone's blood pressure and overall response to exercise very carefully. I would work out on a treadmill or exercise bicycle, then a rowing machine, then join the group of heart patients for weight training. Before or after the exercise sessions, there were also training classes on heart health and healthy eating.

I started to look forward to the cardio fitness training almost immediately. It felt really good to use muscles that I hadn't been using for my many years as an office worker "mouse potato" in front of a computer screen. Not everybody visiting the cardio fitness center felt the same way, though. Some people seemed to feel very defeated by their heart attack experience, as if they had received a death sentence. For those people who had experienced a severe cardiac event or had experienced several events, that was understandable, perhaps.

Fortunately, for me the cardio fitness center was a life sentence, a chance to adopt new attitudes towards my life and to make the most of what I had. The very supportive and encouraging people at the center taught me that paying attention to my health on a regular basis was a good thing. I kept up the cardio fitness sessions three times a week and between those sessions I did a lot of Wii Fit™ exercising, Wii™ sports games and walks with my son. Pretty soon he started to get the exercise "bug" as well! What was good for me was good for him, too.

During my cardio fitness therapy, I made it a point to keep up the pace of this exercise when I was on business trips. On a trip to India, I would exercise on the long airplane trip in a little area at the rear of the cabin. When I got to the hotel, I ran around the room and in the hotel courtyard. On other trips I made it a point to find hotels that had exercise rooms and to keep up my routines. By the time I had finished the cardio fitness training, I had a habit – a good habit. I had gone from being someone who had become afraid to exercise to someone who loved to exercise. I started to feel physically fit for the first time in many, many years. As soon as I left the cardio fitness center I signed up at a local sports club for a membership and kept at my exercise routines four days a week, using the heart rate monitoring equipment recommended to me by the cardio fitness center.

Not surprisingly, with all of this healthy exercise and good eating, I lost weight. In fact, I lost ninety pounds in about nine months, slowly gaining muscle along the way as I was burning off the fat. I had gone from being someone who was dangerously overweight – a heart attack waiting to happen – to someone who was lean and healthy. It was an amazing transition. As I exercised, ate right and got my cholesterol under control, the doctor was able to reduce the amount of some of the medications that I was taking. My body was doing a good job of taking care of itself.

After about a year, I began to gain a bit of weight back, but I wasn't getting fatter. I was starting to put on more muscle but I wasn't looking like a weight-lifter, nor was I trying to look like one. There was simply more of me in "the right places." More importantly, my heart got stronger and stronger. I went from having a kind of gray complexion to a healthy, heart-fed complexion. My whole body had come back to life. In fact, my whole life came back to life. The next summer, when my son and I went out sailing, I noticed right away that I was much more stable and confident raising the sails and working the boat. I was no longer afraid of losing my balance and I was really enjoying the experience again.

Today, my life is so very different than it was before my heart procedure. I make healthy living my highest priority. I now recognize that this is not a selfish thing, but a generous thing. My family needs me to help take care of them, to be alive for them to enjoy the many good times that we have together. My business associates need a healthy "me" if I am also going to be productive for them. If I am not taking care of myself, how can I do that? It may mean saying "no" to some things that aren't good for me, but I have gained the courage to do this consistently, for their sake as well as for my own sake. In the process of doing so, I am passing on good habits to my son. He now has his own exercise routines, and eats more healthily so he will have a longer and better life also. And it's a life that we will enjoy together.

Now, more than three years after my heart attack, my son and I have a lot of fun together. Hopefully I have many happy and healthy years ahead of me with my family, thanks to the miracles that happened in the wake of that fateful day running to catch a train.

I still have to run to catch trains, now and again. And wouldn't you know it: I don't have to worry about it anymore. And neither does my family.

A heart attack turned out to be the event that saved my life. Who would have known?

Over the last three years, I have shared John's success story numerous times with other patients who I thought needed a bit more motivation. What John was able to accomplish in several months of enrollment in the cardiac rehab exercise program is a true testament to John's dedication. It shows the truth of that adage that what you put into a task is what you can expect to get back from it.

One of the benefits of writing and publishing this book is that now I can more easily share John's story in his own words, with so many others, since he is truly an inspiration. John's changes because of his heart attack as the catalyst to those changes are, indeed, encouraging.

However, even though John used his heart attack as a pivotal point to turning his life around, I want to caution those readers who have not yet had a heart attack but who are potentially on the road to one because of lack of exercise, obesity, or other risk factors: Do not wait until you have a heart attack to start yourself on a path to fitness. John was lucky. His first heart attack was a relatively minor one and the somewhat "simple" surgery of implanting stents to open up the blockages in his arteries was 100% successful.

But the dramatic statistics need to be shared about those who suffer a heart attack who are *not* as lucky as John. The harsh reality is that the number of fatalities, as well as long term disabilities, related to a first heart attack are dramatic: The Centers for Disease Control (CDC) reports that by 2009 in the United States, one in every three deaths (about 600,000 annually) was due to cardiovascular disease.[1] What that means is that approximately every 34 seconds, an American will have a coronary event. About every minute, someone will die from one.

The statistics related to disabilities are equally astounding: among an estimated 45 million people in the United States with functional disabilities (the inability to independently perform activities of daily living, such as work, household chores, recreational activities or self-care), heart disease, stroke and high blood pressure are among the 15 leading conditions that caused the disability.[2] According to the Council for Disability Awareness, heart disease (along with cancer and diabetes) cause more disabilities than work-related injuries.[3]

Here are some more statistics that will, it's hoped, inspire you to begin, and not put off, a renewed commitment to your exercise and diet programs, leading to a healthier you: Within six years after a recognized heart attack, 7% of men and 6% of women will experience sudden cardiac death in which the heart stops beating.[2] Brain damage results about four to six minutes after the heart stops pumping blood.[4] Without timely and successful cardiopulmonary resuscitation (CPR), even if the victim survives, the chances of serious disability are great.

If you've had a heart attack already, by all means, use John's heartfelt and powerful story of change as a motivation to do the same for yourself.

But if you are fortunate enough to have not yet had a heart attack, count yourself lucky and consider implementing the heart-healthy exercise routines that you will learn about in this book. Also consider making the diet improvements and following the stress-reduction techniques that you will read about, so you will increase your chances of avoiding a heart attack!

In the next chapter, I'll review heart anatomy so you'll have a better understanding of this pivotal organ. Even if you took biology in high school or college, you might find this review useful. Of course, this information is not meant to be a substitute for the high-level knowledge of your cardiologist, internist or cardiology nurse. It is intended as a general review only.

Chapter 2

Anatomy 101*

The true life story you read in Chapter 1 represents a mere fraction of the numerous heart problems that can have an impact on you. Throughout this book, you will be introduced to various degrees of heart difficulties or complications, numerous tests to provide more information about your heart, and surgical or medication treatments to deal with these conditions. To help you in your understanding of these topics, this chapter provides an overview of what the heart is and what functions it performs in your body.

Your heart is a muscle, and the most important one in your body. It is not a skeletal muscle, such as your shoulders or biceps. These muscles fatigue relatively quickly with any amount of work. Instead, your heart is a specialized cardiac muscle whose job is to pump and contract continuously from the day you're born until the day you die. This is what distinguishes your heart from all other organs in your body. It performs a physical task—pumping, squeezing, contracting—continuously. Your skeletal muscles work only on demand, but your heart is working all the time.

With each contraction, your heart is delivering blood to all of your organs and tissues, including your skeletal muscles, like your shoulders and biceps. The blood is feeding those muscles and organs with all of the oxygen and nutrients required for optimal functioning. With the muscles and organs being fed, your blood has now been depleted of oxygen and nutrients

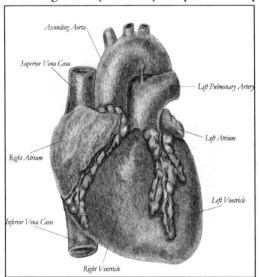

Ascending Aorta

Superior Vena Cava

Left Pulmonary Artery

Left Atrium

Right Atrium

Left Ventricle

Inferior Vena Cava

Right Ventricle

Figure 1. Anterior View of the Heart*

---

* Illustrations are by Tara Macolino. This information is not meant to be a substitute for the high-level expert knowledge of your cardiologist, internist, or cardiology nurse. It is intended as a general review only.

and is immediately sent to your lungs for removal of carbon dioxide and other wastes. This entire process is happening with each heartbeat: about 60 to 100 times per minute!

Your heart is made up of four chambers – the right and left atria, and the right and left ventricles. The atria are the top two smaller chambers that collect blood and pass it over to the bottom chambers, the ventricles. These are the larger chambers that are responsible for greater delivery of blood through the proper pathway.

The right atrium receives deoxygenated blood from large veins called the inferior and superior vena cava. The superior vena cava sends deoxygenated blood from the brain. Meanwhile, the inferior vena cava transports deoxygenated blood from the remainder of the body's tissues.

From the right atrium, the deoxygenated blood passes through a one-way valve called the tricuspid valve and goes to the right ventricle. From there, the blood travels through another one-way valve known as the pulmonic valve. This leads through the pulmonary artery to the right and left lungs for reoxygenation.

The pulmonary artery is one of the two largest arteries in the heart. It contains thick walls made up of elastic tissue. This elasticity enables the arteries to stretch and recoil, which enables blood to propel forward at high pressure into circulation.

This newly oxygenated blood travels through the pulmonary veins and into the left atrium of the heart. From there, it passes through a third one-way valve, the mitral valve, which leads to the left ventricle.

The left ventricle is the largest of the four chambers. This should not be a surprise since its major function is to send this oxygen-rich blood through a fourth one-way valve, the aortic valve, into the aorta and out to all of the various organs and tissues.

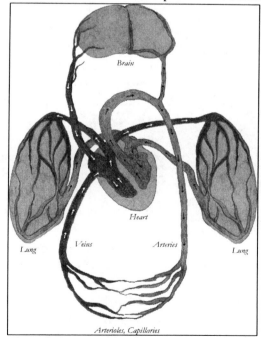

Figure 2. Oxygenated and Deoxygenated Blood Traveling through the Various Chambers of the Heart

The aorta is the largest artery in the heart. Similar to the pulmonary artery, the aorta contains thick, elastic walls which enable the blood to flow to its destinations.

The coronary arteries are smaller arteries contained in the heart muscle itself. Like all other arteries in the body, the coronary arteries supply oxygen-rich blood to a designated area. With coronary arteries, the designated area is in the heart.

The largest of these arteries is the left anterior descending artery (LAD). This is also known as the "widow maker" mainly because blockages in this vessel tend to be more life-threatening. This artery supplies blood to the left atrium and left ventricle.

Since the left ventricle is the largest of the four chambers, this is one chamber you don't want to have a blockage in. The right coronary artery supplies blood to the right atrium and ventricle of the heart. The left coronary artery and circumflex artery supply blood to the posterior regions of the heart.

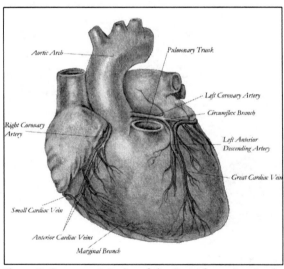

Figure 3. Coronary Arteries of the Heart (anterior view)

Similar to other veins in the body driving oxygen-poor blood back to the heart, the heart contains coronary veins which carry oxygen-poor blood back into the right atrium. The coronary veins in the heart are the small, middle, and great cardiac vein, along with the posterior vein, all of which merge at the coronary sinus and travel into the right atrium. Unlike other veins in the body which send oxygen-poor blood to the superior and inferior vena cava, the blood in the coronary sinus flows directly to the right atrium, bypassing the vena cava.

Another unique characteristic of coronary blood flow is that when the heart muscle relaxes, the oxygen-rich blood is carried through the coronary arteries to its designated areas. For the rest of the body, oxygen-rich blood is carried when the heart muscle contracts.

When we partake in physical activity such as exercise, a large percentage of this oxygen-rich blood is being shuttled to our starving skeletal muscles in order to keep working. This particular function of the heart muscle helps explain why you have been warned as a kid not to go swimming right after eating. Because such a large amount of oxygen-rich blood is required for the exercising muscles, less is available for the organs responsible for digestion, such as the stomach. As a result, digestion is slowed.

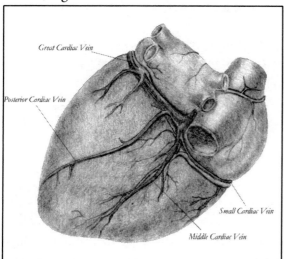

Figure 4. Coronary Veins of the Heart (posterior view)

Another interesting fact is that just as a greater percentage of oxygen-rich blood travels to the skeletal muscles, a similar amount of deoxygenated blood travels back to the heart at a greater rate, decreasing the workload of the heart. This is one of the numerous benefits of exercise to the heart. (Additional benefits of exercise for your heart will be covered in later chapters.)

This whole blood-redistribution process happens in less than one second. The contractions of the atria and ventricles indicate a single heart beat. An average heart rate is 60-100 beats per minute (bpm). With such a huge responsibility, it is important to do what you can to ensure your heart's proper functioning. In upcoming chapters, you will learn the consequences of a less-than-optimally functioning heart.

Chapter 3

Heart-related Illnesses, Tests and Treatments

Now that you have a better understanding of the anatomy and proper functioning of the heart, we will learn what results when the heart is no longer functioning at an optimal level.

Let's begin by addressing various heart-related illnesses and arrhythmias. I will then describe some of the more common testing procedures to diagnose these conditions. This chapter concludes with a discussion of current treatment options for those heart conditions.

HEART-RELATED ILLNESSES

Myocardial Infarction (MI)

Coronary atherosclerosis involves the accumulation of lipids and fibrous plaques within the coronary arteries. These plaques cause a narrowing of the vessels, which leads to myocardial ischemia. This is simply a lack of oxygen-rich blood flowing to an area of the heart muscle. Ischemia lasting more than an hour causes irreversible cellular damage and cell death. The result is an acute myocardial infarction (MI) or heart attack.

Classic signs and symptoms of MI include:

- chest pressure or pain that may radiate to the arms, neck, upper back, or jaw
- nausea
- vomiting
- sweating
- increased cardiac enzymes seen on a blood test
- specific EKG changes

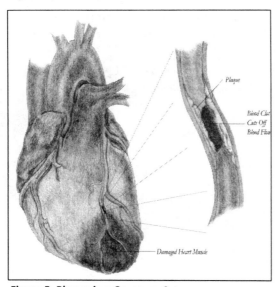

Plaque

Blood Clot
Cuts Off
Blood Flow

Damaged Heart Muscle

Figure 5. Plaque in a Coronary Artery

Those who have an MI can have just one of these signs or nearly all present.

It is important to note that those who are experiencing an MI can have "non-classic" signs or symptoms, including generalized fatigue, shortness of breath, sleep disturbance and anxiety. Such symptoms tend to be more prevalent in women. Unfortunately, those symptoms are often ignored or misdiagnosed.

An MI usually affects the left ventricle and the ability of the large chambers of the heart to contract efficiently. This is apparent in the area of deadened tissue. The extent of the damage, as well as the degree of myocardial ischemia, determines the risk of future cardiovascular morbidity and mortality.

Ejection fraction, defined as the percentage of blood pumped out of the left ventricle with each beat, is one parameter to determine the degree of ventricular dysfunction. A normal ejection fraction is $62 \pm 6\%$. This is measured at rest, with an ultrasound of the heart, a device that is called an echocardiogram.[1]

Valvular Heart Disease

Valvular heart disease is a very broad term that can relate to one or more of four major valves in the heart. These are the aortic valve, pulmonic valve, bicuspid, and tricuspid valve. The symptoms, limitations and treatment options vary, depending on which valves are involved, whether the valves are stenotic (failing to open adequately) or regurgitant (with backward flow or leaking of blood), the severity of the valve lesions, and the presence of preexisting dysfunction or disease.

With mitral stenosis, there is an inability of the mitral valve to open adequately. As the valve area decreases, there is increased pressure between the left atrium and left ventricle. As this pressure increases, pulmonary vascular pressure increases, resulting in shortness of breath. Initially, this shortness of breath occurs at lower levels of activity. Shortness of breath at rest and pulmonary edema (swelling and/or fluid accumulation in the lungs) are other common symptoms of valvular heart disease.

Typical symptoms include:
- shortness of breath
- chest pain
- hoarseness
- coughing up blood
- infective endocarditis (infection of the inner lining of the heart). If left untreated, it can damage and destroy heart vessels.

An echocardiogram is usually done to evaluate the size of the left atrium, so as to determine the mitral valve area as well as the course of action to take.

Surgical correction is indicated when physical activity is substantially limited. Usually severe symptoms develop when the mitral valve area is <1.0 cm^2.[2]

With mitral valve regurgitation, there is a backward flow or leaking of blood between the left atrium and left ventricle. Normally, there is a one-way valve preventing back flow. If blood is not adequately pumped in the forward direction but is flowing back in the reverse direction, a less-than-adequate percentage of oxygen-rich blood is available to supply organs and tissues. But when problems occur with the mitral valve, or with preexisting diseases or infection, the mitral valve fails to function properly, which could result in this condition.

Symptoms depend on the rate of development and severity of the regurgitation. Symptoms may not present themselves until the left ventricle begins to fail. Someone with this condition may even be asymptomatic, experiencing such discomforts as fatigue and shortness of breath, but by the time they do, irreversible dysfunction of the ventricle often has developed.

Like mitral valve stenosis, mitral valve regurgitation is discovered with an echocardiogram. Angiography (x-ray exam of blood vessels and heart chambers) is another test done to determine the severity of mitral valve regurgitation and to see if bypass surgery is necessary.

Aortic stenosis is common in older people (ages 65 and up), usually the result of years of normal stress on the valves and by calcification (accumulation of hard deposits of calcium salts). People in their 70s will commonly develop symptoms such as angina, shortness of breath and/or dizziness. Without surgical intervention, people with aortic stenosis can expect to live only another two to five years from the onset of symptoms.[2] Therefore, aortic valve repair or replacement is usually necessary. Similar to the mitral valve, an echocardiogram can determine the severity of the stenosis.

Aortic regurgitation is another possibility affecting the aortic valve. This is similar to mitral regurgitation, except it occurs within the aortic valve. Those with this condition tend to show symptoms such as shortness

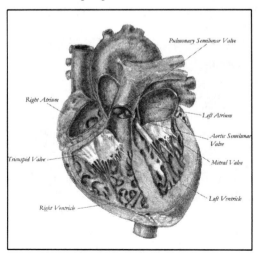

Figure 6. The Four Valves of the Heart

of breath with exertion during their 40's and 50's. When these symptoms develop, irreversible left ventricular dysfunction may have occurred. Thus, it is important that these people are followed closely with an echocardiogram to show the severity of the regurgitation and to determine if and when surgery is required. Aortic valve repair or replacement surgery is typically necessary when the left ventricle becomes dilated, due to mitral valve regurgitation or when significant symptoms develop.

As with mitral stenosis, tricuspid stenosis can occur. In fact, some mitral valve diseases often coexist. People usually complain of fatigue, as well as swelling of the abdomen and lower extremities. Significant fluid retention and distended neck veins are usually present.

As with the other forms of valvular heart disease, an echocardiogram is used to diagnose and determine the cause and severity. Surgical repair is the treatment of choice and is usually done at the same time as mitral valve surgery.

Tricuspid regurgitation is commonly caused by enlargement of the right ventricle, but can result from a number of different diseases and disorders. If pulmonary hypertension (high pulmonary artery pressure) is absent, this condition is usually tolerated well. If pulmonary hypertension exists, edema and fatigue develop. With an echocardiogram, the pressure and severity of the regurgitation is determined, as well as the pressure of the right ventricle. Narrowing of the tricuspid annulus (ring-shaped structure) with a prosthesis called a carpentier ring can improve the regurgitation. In general, no surgical intervention is required for this condition alone.

Similar to aortic stenosis and regurgitation, the pulmonic valve can experience stenosis and regurgitation. Pulmonic stenosis is often congenital, while regurgitation is caused by dilation of the pulmonary artery or valve ring, related to pulmonary hypertension. Symptoms of pulmonic stenosis are usually absent with mild stenosis. As it becomes more severe, symptoms include heart failure, dizziness, shortness of breath with exertion, and chest pain. Any symptoms that occur with pulmonic regurgitation have to do with the underlying cause.

> *The role of exercise: People with significant pulmonic stenosis should avoid vigorous physical activity, due to the high risk of fainting. Again, an echocardiogram is used to determine the presence, cause and significance of the lesions.*

CHF (congestive heart failure)

Congestive heart failure (CHF) is a disorder in which the heart muscle is unable to effectively pump oxygen-rich blood to the various tissues of the body. This is usually due to the loss of heart muscle related to an MI or a decrease in the left ventricle's ability to contract.

With an inability of the ventricle to contract and pump out blood efficiently, there tends to be a problem with blood filling the chamber. As a result, a less-than-adequate percentage of oxygen-rich blood is available to supply the organs and tissues.

Without adequate oxygen-rich blood flow to the tissues, serious problems can result. One problem is that the skeletal muscle metabolism will be impaired. When we exercise, blood flow is enhanced to the exercising muscle. If our hearts are unable to deliver enough oxygen-rich blood to the exercising muscles, fatigue will set in relatively quickly. This results in a reduced exercise tolerance. With inadequate perfusion (blood flow) to the kidneys, sodium and water retention can result. Furthermore, the backflow of blood due to the inability of the left ventricle to pump blood can lead to right-sided heart failure.

Classic signs of CHF include:
- fluid retention
- fatigue
- shortness of breath

Initial treatment of CHF involves finding and treating the underlying cause. Medications are a second line of treatment that can help reduce symptoms.

The role of exercise: In the past, exercise was discouraged for those with CHF for fear that it would cause further harm to an already-weakened heart. But more recent studies have shown increases in exercise capacity after exercise training in those with heart failure. Improvements seem to be related to skeletal muscle adaptation, as opposed to cardiac changes.[2] Nevertheless, exercise training programs are effective in decreasing CHF symptoms and enhancing the ability to sustain low-level activities.[2] This can greatly enhance the quality of these people's lives.

Exercise has been proven to be a valuable adjunct to other modes of treatment.

It is important to note that health status with CHF can change very quickly. Those with CHF should be alert for rapid changes in weight and/or blood pressure, worsened shortness of breath, angina with exertion, or increased arrhythmias. Those with CHF are at an increased risk of sudden death and should not hesitate to inform their cardiologist of a worsening of their symptoms.

Common Arrhythmias

The following information will help explain some of the more common arrhythmias you or your loved ones may be subject to, especially anyone who has preexisting heart disease. Although this information will not teach you how to read and interpret EKGs, it will increase your awareness of these arrhythmias. As a result, you may better recognize signs or symptoms that may occur, and take appropriate action.

EKGs are a tracing of the electrical activity of the heart. In a perfect world, our resting EKG should show what is called normal sinus rhythm. This occurs when the natural pacemaker of the heart (sinoatrial node or SA node) generates an electrical impulse in the right atrium, causing both atria to contract. This is represented by a P wave. This electrical impulse travels downward through several structures in the heart and stimulates a contraction of both left and right ventricles (Fig. 7a). This is represented by a QRS complex (Fig. 7b). It's the PQRS complex which symbolizes an actual heart beat on an EKG tracing.

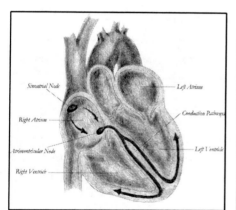

**Figure 7(a). The SA Node
Generating an Electrical Impulse**

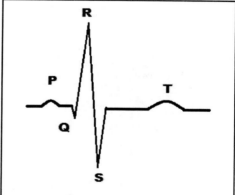

**Figure 7(b). An Example of a
PQRST Complex of an EKG**

Normal Sinus Rhythm

During the contraction of these ventricles, the atria are already filling with blood, waiting for the next impulse to be generated. After the ventricles contract, pumping blood throughout the body, they quickly start to fill, anticipating the next electrical impulse. The T wave represents repolarization, where the heart cells regain their energy to be stimulated again. This whole process happens in milliseconds. The heart rate with normal sinus rhythm is 60-100 bpm.

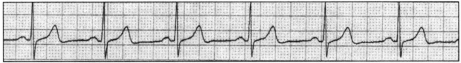

Figure 8: Normal Sinus Rhythm

Sinus Tachycardia

A couple of different circumstances may exist in which it is normal to have a rhythm other than normal sinus rhythm. For example, when exercising, it is not unusual to have a heart rate greater than 100 bpm. Sinus tachycardia is the name given to the rhythm in which the SA node tells the atria to beat faster than 100 bpm, which causes the ventricles to do the same. To be exact, the heart rate in sinus tachycardia is 100-150 bpm. This is a perfectly normal response to exercise, or sometimes when mentally stimulated, such as with anxiety, fear or panic. In some people, it may be "normal" for them to have a resting heart rate in the low 100's (i.e. 102 bpm). Technically, this would be referred to as sinus tachycardia.

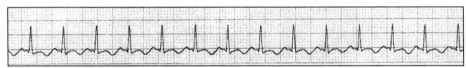

Figure 9: Sinus Tachycardia

Sinus Bradycardia

Sinus bradycardia is the name given to the rhythm that is less than 60 bpm. The SA node still initiates the beat; hence the name "sinus." This rhythm may present itself as a result of certain medications, such as beta blockers. In well-conditioned athletes, such as marathon runners, a resting heart rate in the 50s could be normal. No intervention would be necessary for this. For those who normally are not that low, especially if symptomatic (i.e. fatigue, dizziness, fainting), seeking medical assistance should take priority.

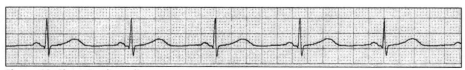

Figure 10: Sinus Bradycardia

Atrial Fibrillation

Atrial fibrillation is one of the more common arrhythmias. In those who have recently had a CABG (coronary artery bypass grafting), it is the most common arrhythmia, one in which the SA node is no longer the pacemaker of the heart. Instead, multiple parts of the atria contract in a continuous, rapid-firing manner. Only an occasional impulse gets through to the ventricles to cause a contraction. This produces an irregular ventricular rhythm which means an irregular heart rate.

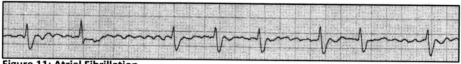

Figure 11: Atrial Fibrillation

You can have what's called "controlled" atrial fibrillation where the heart rate falls between the 60's and low 100's. "Uncontrolled" atrial fibrillation is where the heart rate is out of the "normal" range. You may have a resting heart rate in the 130's, for example. Under such conditions, medications such as calcium channel blockers are often prescribed to help control the heart rate.

Speaking of medications, whether you have controlled or uncontrolled atrial fibrillation, a blood thinner, such as Coumadin,* is usually prescribed to reduce the risk of a stroke. That is because those with atrial fibrillation are at a very high risk of a stroke, due to the ineffective passage of blood flow from atrium to ventricles. Just as we can develop blockages in our coronary arteries, resulting in a heart attack, we can also form blockages in arteries nourishing the brain, leading to a "brain attack" (or stroke).

A stroke occurs when oxygen-rich blood is unable to reach a part of the brain due to a major blockage or bleed. In this case, blood that is unable to flow from atria to ventricles can form clots. This can lead to a blockage of blood flow to the brain. If the compromised area of the brain does not receive nourishment within several hours and interventions such as medication and surgery are unsuccessful, if the victim survives, he or she can be left with a mental and/or physical disability (i.e. difficulty in pronouncing words, memory loss, weakness, paralysis).

There are three types of atrial fibrillation: *paroxysmal atrial fibrillation; persistent atrial fibrillation; or permanent atrial fibrillation.*

- *Paroxysmal atrial fibrillation* is of sudden onset and temporary form. It usually lasts less than seven days.
- *Persistent atrial fibrillation* lasts longer than seven days.

- *Permanent atrial fibrillation* is the name given to the type in which electrical cardioversion (shocking the heart out of the arrhythmia) is unsuccessful.

Many of those with atrial fibrillation have no symptoms and may not know they are in it. But for those who do experience symptoms, here are the most common ones:
- fatigue
- shortness of breath with exertion
- dizziness, especially with a lower or higher heart rate such as with uncontrolled atrial fibrillation.

There are several ways to try to get someone out of atrial fibrillation. In some cases, those with this condition can break the rhythm without any intervention. In other cases, medical intervention may be attempted.

At this time, there is no cure for atrial fibrillation. Attempts are made to simply control or eliminate it.

The type of intervention selected to eliminate or control atrial fibrillation is dependent upon which type of atrial fibrillation the person has.

One intervention is pharmacological therapy. An anti-arrhythmic drug, such as Amiodarone˙, may be successful in breaking the rhythm. But this drug may not be suitable for some people due to potentially undesirable side effects. Potential side effects include:
- vision changes (blurred vision, seeing halos, vision loss)
- respiratory problems (wheezing, fibrosis – damage and scarring of the lungs)
- absence of taste or smell
- nausea
- vomiting
- loss of appetite
- insomnia

If the medication is unsuccessful or contraindicated, electrical cardioversion is another option. This is where the individual is "shocked" with defibrillation pads at a low energy level, such as 30 joules (200-360 joules are given for cardiac arrest). This may be enough to break the arrhythmia.[3]

But if neither option is successful, other nonsurgical and surgical interventions exist. One such option is nonsurgical ablation, a procedure in which a catheter is inserted from the groin, arm or neck area into a specific area of the heart, primarily around the pulmonary veins. A special machine directs energy from the catheter to that "excitable" area of the heart causing this arrhythmia, and basically *zaps* it so the arrhythmia can no longer occur at that point. As a result, it will cease firing. The natural pacemaker now has the opportunity to take over, initiating a stronger, more efficient atrial contraction. This procedure is done by an electrophysiologist, a cardiologist who specializes in the electrical activity of the heart. It is a minimally invasive procedure, which leads to a quick recovery. The chest remains closed and the heart continues to beat.

Surgical ablation is another treatment option that is used to remedy atrial fibrillation; it can be either a minimally invasive or "open" surgery. The Maze procedure is one of the surgical interventions. It has been used since 1987 and has undergone two major modifications since that time. The Cox-III Maze procedure is a highly complex and invasive procedure. It involves a thoracotomy, where the breast bone is cut and ribs are spread. It targets the left and right upper chamber mechanisms, and it has produced an impressive success rate in eliminating atrial fibrillation.[4] The cardiac surgeon basically "cuts" the "bad" tissue out. Due to the invasiveness of the procedure, numerous risks are involved and recovery can be difficult. As a result, not everyone with atrial fibrillation would be a suitable candidate.

The Cox-IV Maze procedure is similar to Cox-III but differs in that instead of cutting the "bad" tissue, it ablates it.

The main problem with this treatment is there's a questionable reduction in dependability. There can be an electrical "reconnection" in which the arrhythmia can return or persist due to the presence of enough sensitive tissue.

A mini-Maze procedure is a minimally invasive option which doesn't involve any large incisions or opening of the chest wall. Three to four small incisions are made on each side of the chest. A thoracoscope is then inserted to view the heart while an ablation device is inserted to "zap" the target tissue. Although it is said to be minimally invasive, the lungs have to be collapsed to get them out of the way. This could easily cause complications, especially postoperatively. This is an option suitable for those with paroxysmal atrial fibrillation and/or early forms of atrial fibrillation. It will focus on the sensitive tissue around the pulmonary veins but won't address the back wall of the chambers.

One of the more recent additions to the list of surgical options is the convergent hybrid procedure. It can treat more advanced stages of atrial fibrillation by accessing a greater amount of atrial tissue. It is far less invasive with no disturbance to the lungs, no breast-bone cutting or rib spreading, and involves only a small abdominal incision. The procedure is performed by both a cardiac surgeon and electrophysiologist. In this way, both the mechanical and electrical flaws of the heart are addressed. The success rate appears to be about 80%. It's important to point out again that the procedure is not appropriate for all types of atrial fibrillation.

With many of these surgical interventions, there is a 10- to 12-week period where a patient could still be in atrial fibrillation. This is known as the "Blinking Period." It doesn't necessarily mean the surgery was a failure. It just might be taking some time to permanently be out of the arrhythmia. At this time, no exact cause for this delay after surgery is known.

Despite all of these interventions, a good number of people live their lives comfortably in atrial fibrillation. Risks and benefits of each option need to be weighed. Of course, if you have atrial fibrillation, it is best to discuss what options might be best in your case with your cardiologist.

Those who remain in the arrhythmia are usually on calcium channel blockers to control their heart rate, as well as blood thinners to reduce their risk of stroke. The important thing to realize is the value of following your doctor's orders when it comes to taking medications which, in the case of Coumadin will require regular blood work to make sure what is known as an INR rate is within an acceptable range. INR stands for international normalized ratio and measures the time it takes for blood to clot and compares it to an average. A therapeutic INR is usually considered to be 2.0 to 3.5 depending on the clinical situation. It may also be advised to eat a diet that is low in vitamin K because vitamin K can increase the clotting factors in the blood. Also, be aware of the onset of new symptoms, such as shortness of breath, rapid heart rate or dizziness, which may indicate a worsening of the condition.

Supraventricular Tachycardia
This is another arrhythmia that can occur, especially in those with coronary artery disease. Supraventricular tachycardia (SVT) is an arrhythmia in which the electrical impulse originates anywhere above the ventricles. The heart rate is greater than 150 bpm. It could present itself as just a sudden initiation that breaks on its own, called paroxysmal (sudden) supraventricular tachycardia. It could also be of longer duration that doesn't break on its own, and would require a pharmacological intervention.

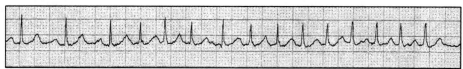

Figure 12: Supraventricular Tachycardia

Similar to atrial fibrillation, people with SVT may initially not be aware that they have this condition. But by simply checking their pulse, they would realize that this rapid heart rate is not normal. Symptoms of SVT include:

- lightheadedness
- fainting
- chest pain

SVT is an arrhythmia that needs to get treatment. Going to an emergency department for medical management is essential. Vagal maneuvers (techniques that stimulate the vagus nerve) such as gagging, holding your breath and bearing down, or coughing may be enough to break this arrhythmia. Similar to atrial fibrillation, electrical cardioversion may be done if all other attempts to manage this arrhythmia fail.

Premature Atrial Contractions

A premature atrial contraction (PAC) is an electrical impulse that appears in the atrium, but earlier than when the SA node (natural pacemaker of the heart) would fire. This impulse "beats out" the SA node. The heart rhythm would be regular, except for the extra beat. Because this other atrial contraction occurs, a normal ventricular contraction would follow.

PACs are generally harmless. People are usually asymptomatic. They may be aware of an occasional extra heartbeat if measuring their pulse but the only way to truly identify PACs is with an EKG machine. For some people with frequent PACs, it can be a precursor to developing atrial fibrillation.

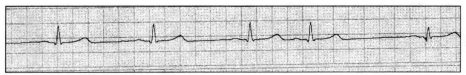

Figure 13: Premature Atrial Contraction

Premature Ventricular Contractions

Premature ventricular contractions (PVCs) are similar to PACs in that they occur spontaneously, cause an irregular heart rate, and prevent the SA node from generating the electrical impulse. When a PVC occurs, the pacemaker of the heart becomes one originating somewhere in the ventricles. This is usually harmless, especially if it occurs infrequently. Healthy individuals may actually get a PVC from time to time. It becomes a problem if it becomes more frequent, especially if grouped together. Two PVCs in a row is called a couplet. Three in a row is considered ventricular tachycardia. This can become more serious, especially if it becomes prolonged. PVCs can occur as a result of certain medications, electrolyte imbalances, or simply due to trauma to the heart (i.e. CABG, PTCA, etc.). Similar to PACs, the only way to know you have them is by having your EKG rhythm interpreted.

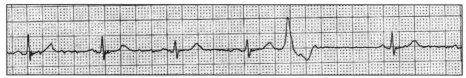

Figure 14: Premature Ventricular Contraction

Ventricular Tachycardia

Ventricular tachycardia is defined as a series of three or more PVCs. It could be a sudden run that breaks on its own or keeps going which would require swift medical treatment. With ventricular tachycardia, a pacemaker in the ventricle becomes irritable and fires rapidly. The heart rate is generally between 150-250 bpm. Although the atria are still contracting at their own rate, the larger ventricles are taking over and initiating the rapid heartbeat. If this is a sudden occurrence that breaks on its own, you wouldn't really know that this was the specific arrhythmia, unless your EKG rhythm was monitored, as in a cardiac rehabilitation program. With this occurrence, a cardiologist must be notified. If the ventricular tachycardia did not break on its own, the individual would need to be hospitalized as soon as possible for treatment.

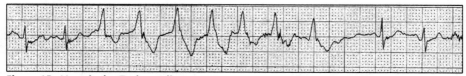

Figure 15 : Ventricular Tachycardia

The person with ventricular tachycardia may or may not be symptomatic. Symptoms could range between lightheadedness, fatigue and shortness of breath, and end up with unconsciousness.

Ventricular tachycardia is a very serious arrhythmia. The ventricles can handle the rapid heart rate for only so long. If untreated, the ventricles will eventually become exhausted. Cardiac arrest and death may result.

Treatment for ventricular tachycardia would include anti-arrhythmic medication and possibly defibrillation. A good rule of thumb to follow is if you check your pulse at rest and find it to be rapid (i.e. roughly 150 bpm or greater), do not hesitate to call 911, regardless of how you feel. By the time symptoms appear, it may be too late to react.

TESTS

The following overview will provide you with general information on various tests your cardiologist may suggest. Some of these tests you may already be familiar with. Others you may have never heard of. It's not a bad idea to become familiar with the different tests that exist. You never know if you or a loved one will need one of them at some point. Having an idea of what to expect should help decrease anxiety and possibly help your performance during the test, which may lead to collecting more accurate data.

The Bruce Maximal Graded Exercise Stress Test
When a cardiologist sends you for an exercise stress test, commonly called "a stress test," it is usually done on a treadmill, following what is known as the Bruce Protocol. The Bruce Protocol is a test which starts out as a walking test and becomes a running test by the fourth stage.[5,6]
Subjects are hooked up to a 12-lead EKG. An IV is inserted, where a radioactive dye is administered. This is used for nuclear imagery, done before and after the exercise.

Those taking this test will start out at 1.7 mph at a 10% incline for three minutes. EKG is continuously measured. Heart rate and blood pressure are monitored at each stage, as well as rate of perceived exertion (RPE). (RPE will be discussed further in a later chapter).

After three minutes, Stage 2 begins with an increase to 2.5 mph at a 12% incline. After three minutes, Stage 3 begins with 3.4 mph and a 14% incline. After another three minutes, Stage 4 begins with 4.2 mph and a 16% incline. By this time, the subject is running (if he or she even makes it this far).

The purpose of this stress test is to bring the subject's heart rate to near-maximum, monitoring the EKG closely and checking for abnormal perfusion (blood flow) throughout the coronary arteries. Subjects are asked to inform the technologist about one minute before needing to stop. A radioactive dye is injected at this time.

The test will be terminated if:

1. The subject requests to stop.
2. The systolic blood pressure drops more than 10 mmHg with increasing workloads (especially if other evidence of poor perfusion exists).
3. The heart rate fails to rise with increasing workloads.
4. EKG changes indicate ischemia.
5. Other symptoms occur, such as moderately severe angina or dizziness, or the subject becomes pale.

The subject can expect to stay at the testing site for several hours. Nuclear imaging is done after the exercise when the subject is lying down. Not only is this stress test valuable for revealing perfusion abnormalities, it will also show how "fit" the subject is. As a clinical exercise physiologist, I often use the results of a stress test in writing an individual's exercise prescription. It is therefore beneficial to have the subject give his or her best effort on the treadmill for the most accurate data. For those who are not in very good shape, for whom the stress test might be too exhausting to attempt, alternative protocols can be used for a more gradual increase in intensity.

Stress Echocardiogram
A stress echocardiogram is an echocardiogram combined with an exercise EKG to increase the accuracy of a stress test, as well as to determine how much of the heart may be at risk, due to ischemia (lack of oxygen-rich blood). Echocardiographic studies at rest are compared with others immediately after treadmill exercise. Images need to be obtained within the first two minutes after exercise because abnormal heart wall motion tends to normalize beyond this point. Advantages of a stress echocardiogram over nuclear imaging include cheaper cost, a shorter test, and no exposure to low-level ionizing radiation.

Exercise Nuclear Imaging
With exercise nuclear imaging, a radioactive dye is administered with images of the heart obtained within 30-60 minutes. Exercise or a pharmacologically induced stress test is done one to three hours later. The dye is administered again one minute before exercise concludes. Stress images are then obtained 30-60 minutes after dye administration. Comparing resting images with stress

images help determine whether any perfusion abnormalities are new (blockages seen under stress) or old (blockages seen at rest, possibly related to old MI or previous heart damage). The images are displayed in a manner which shows the heart in three dimensions. This enhances the ability to detect blockages.

There are several drawbacks to this kind of test. It is expensive, especially since additional equipment and personnel are required to run it. A nuclear technician is needed to administer the dye and take the pictures. A physician trained in nuclear medicine is needed to interpret the pictures. Another drawback is the fact that the subject is exposed to low-level ionizing radiation. Nevertheless, it is a test that is commonly used and it provides fairly accurate data.

Pharmacological Stress Test

Many people are not candidates for exercise stress testing, such as those in poor physical shape, those with orthopedic or neurological issues, and those with peripheral vascular disease. Pharmacological stress testing is a suitable alternative for such individuals. It is used to establish a diagnosis of coronary artery disease, assess the prognosis after a heart attack or in chronic angina, and determine the cardiac risk in those preparing for surgery.

The test involves infusing an IV medication to gradually increase the heart rate. This will also increase the heart's demand for oxygen-rich blood. The dose is increased until a maximum is given or the testing endpoint is achieved. If the endpoint is not achieved, a second type of medicine is infused to further increase the heart rate. Endpoints include serious arrhythmias or other EKG changes indicating ischemia, angina, significant increase or decrease in blood pressure, intolerable side effects, or if an adequate heart rate was achieved. Heart rate, blood pressure and EKG are measured throughout the test, as well as echocardiographic images obtained.

In addition to a medicine that increases heart rate, a vasodilator (medicine that opens up the arteries) is also commonly used. This would cause "normal" arteries to open up but not stenotic ones. As a result, you'd see increased blood flow to the "normal" arteries and decreased blood flow to the stenotic ones.

Cardiac Catheterization

A cardiac catheterization is a study in which a catheter is inserted into an artery or vein and guided into the heart. A contrast dye is injected to help explore the structure and functioning of the heart. Information about oxygen saturation and pressure readings within heart chambers can be obtained from this procedure.[7] The decision to do an angioplasty or bypass surgery is commonly made based on information obtained from a catheterization. EKG monitoring is done throughout the procedure. Patients are instructed to refrain from foods and fluids for anywhere from six to 18 hours before the procedure. Local anesthesia is used. A feeling of warmth and fluttering sensation in the heart are commonly felt. The procedure may be contraindicated in those with iodine sensitivity and/or kidney problems. After the procedure, it is important to check the injection site for swelling and bleeding, as well as checking color, sensation and pulses of the extremity.

PET Scan

A positron emission tomography (PET) scan is an imaging test that can detect changes in organs and certain tissues early, often before diseases progress. PET scans can detect areas of decreased blood flow in the heart, and can differentiate dead heart muscle from poorly-functioning heart muscle that may benefit from a procedure such as a CABG or angioplasty. It can also be used for neurological diseases, cancer, infection, and certain inflammatory diseases.

A radioactive substance is used, similar to nuclear stress tests. The radioactive substance is administered via IV. In 30-60 minutes, the exam is started with the subject lying still. The exam lasts 30-45 minutes. If heart disease is suspected, a PET scan could be combined with a stress test, which could last a few hours.

The unique characteristic of PET scanning is that unlike other scans it doesn't show structural detail of the organ. What it does show is the chemical activity of the organs or tissues. Images of more or less intense color will tell if the organ is functioning at a high or low level.

Holter Monitor

A Holter monitor is a portable EKG device, used to record the electrical activity of the heart for an extended period of time. It is named after its inventor, Dr. Norman Holter. Anywhere from three to eight EKG leads are positioned on the person, along with a small box attached to the patient's belt. Most record EKG for 24 hours. Others record activity for 30 days.

The main objective of the Holter monitor is to detect cardiac arrhythmias that would be difficult to identify in a shorter period of time. For those with symptoms that come and go quickly, a 30-day recorder is a useful tool.

In addition to wearing the monitor, patients are usually asked to keep a diary of activities, as well as to record times that symptoms occur, such as unusual fatigue, lightheadedness, rapid heart rate, and palpitations. Doctors can then match the EKG at the time that symptoms occur to what the patient was doing at that time.

We will now turn to the most common treatments for the main heart conditions that we have discussed so far, such as atrial fibrillation and other serious arrhythmias, myocardial infarction, and CHF. If you or a loved one have been diagnosed with any of these, read on.

TREATMENTS

CABG

Coronary Artery Bypass Grafting (CABG) is a surgical technique in which a blood vessel, usually a saphenous vein in the leg or internal mammary artery in the chest, is used to bypass a clogged coronary artery. The goals with CABG are to increase oxygen-rich blood flow, thus providing nourishment to the area of the heart with the blocked vessel, and to potentially reduce cardiovascular morbidity and mortality. CABG is used to relieve symptoms of angina that aren't relieved with medication. It is also used to preserve left ventricular function in those with already compromised left ventricular functioning, with significant additional heart muscle at risk, due to existing coronary artery disease. CABG is also used when other interventions, such as an angioplasty, are contraindicated.

People who undergo CABG tend to be older (over 60 years of age), with significant blockages, such as triple-vessel disease and a poor ejection fraction. The average ejection fraction in a person undergoing CABG is 38%. The patency of the graft tends to be greater in those who have the internal mammary gland used, as opposed to the saphenous vein.

CABG is not without its share of complications. There is always the risk of blockage of the new graft. During surgery, patients are at risk of developing an MI. Advanced age (75 years of age or more) poses greater risks.

Observation and monitoring of those undergoing CABG during exercise-based cardiac rehabilitation can help detect deterioration in health status. Several possibilities are recurring angina, lightheadedness or dysrhythmias.

People recovering from CABG will have a surgical incision down the middle of the chest in the mid-sternal area. To allow complete healing, upper body exercises such as the rowing machine, as well as heavy weight training, should be avoided for the first 12 weeks after surgery.

PTCA

Percutaneous transluminal coronary angioplasty (PTCA) is another revascularization technique, used to compress and redistribute plaque as well as stretch the vessel wall to increase its diameter. This will help increase blood flow by basically unclogging the clogged artery.

In PTCA, a balloon catheter is directed to the clogged site. The balloon inflates at the area that is clogged, which produces the desired effect. A stent is often used to keep the lumen patent and to help reduce the risk of clogging up again. There are two types of stents often used – bare metal stents and drug-elluding stents. Neither type is without risk of re-stenosis (clogging up again). In fact, roughly 30-40% of individuals undergoing PTCA will develop re-stenosis of the treated artery within six months of the procedure.[2]

Compared to CABG with a hospital stay of six to nine days, those with PTCA are usually discharged within a day or two. With a quicker recovery period, PTCA tends to be the revascularization method of choice. More than half of those diagnosed with ischemic heart disease, where there is a blockage in one or more vessels, undergo PTCA.[2]

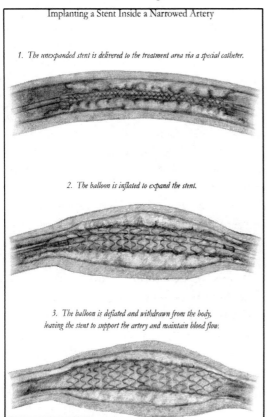

Implanting a Stent Inside a Narrowed Artery

1. *The unexpanded stent is delivered to the treatment area via a special catheter.*

2. *The balloon is inflated to expand the stent.*

3. *The balloon is deflated and withdrawn from the body, leaving the stent to support the artery and maintain blood flow.*

Figure 16. Placement of a Stent in a Clogged Artery

Those recovering from PTCA can begin to resume normal activities, including light to moderate exercise within the first couple of days after the procedure. Similar to CABG, those recovering from PTCA would benefit from an exercise-based cardiac rehabilitation program with close monitoring and supervision. This way, signs and symptoms of re-stenosis can be detected early, which improves the chances of a favorable outcome.

Unlike CABG patients, those with PTCA do not have the same upper body restrictions, since no mid-sternal incision exists. For a couple of weeks, they will have to watch their groin area where the balloon catheter was inserted for the possibility of hematoma or infection. Flying in an airplane should be avoided for several months after the PTCA. For unknown reasons, the air pressure at such high elevation can cause complications with the stent. It would be best to check with your cardiologist before flying.

Pacemakers and AICDs

For optimal functioning of the heart muscle, the filling of the atria and ventricles have to be adequate and synchronized. In addition, they need to contract efficiently in order to pump an adequate amount of blood throughout the body. If this functioning is flawed, significant symptoms can occur at rest and during exercise. In such circumstances, some forms of cardiac pacing may be warranted, requiring a pacemaker. In those with certain serious dysrhythmias occurring at the ventricles, a device known as an automated implantable cardioverter defibrillator (AICD) may be warranted.

A typical pacemaker consists of one or two leads and a pulse generator. Leads can be inserted into your right atrium, right ventricle, or both. These leads are connected to the pulse generator which is positioned near the clavicle. The job of these leads is to sense and pace. In order to sense, electrical signals from the heart need to be received. If no such signal is received, the pacemaker will fire, causing the atria or ventricles to contract.

Different types of pacemakers exist and are classified according to which chambers of the heart are sensed and/or paced, when scarring responses are inhibited, as well as a rate-responsiveness programming. A rate-responsiveness programming provides a heart rate adjustment, based on the body's metabolic needs. For example, the pacemaker will provide an appropriate increase in heart rate in response to various stimuli, such as greater respiratory rate, increased blood temperature, and amplified muscular activity (e.g. exercise).

In those at risk for life-threatening ventricular dysrhythmias, AICDs are sometimes used to electrically terminate them. An AICD consists of a lead system and a cardioverter defibrillator. The leads track the heart rhythm and send information to the pulse generator. When one of these life-threatening dysrhythmias occurs, it is detected by the unit and preprogrammed therapies are sent back to terminate the dysrhythmia. The dysrhythmia can be pace-terminated, or if severe enough, an electrical cardioversion shock can be delivered.

AICDs do not come without risks. Those with AICDs are at risk for receiving inappropriate shocks with exercise. This can result if a person's heart rate with exercise exceeds the heart rate programmed in the AICD to deliver a shock.

A dysrhythmia may also occur with exercise that can mimic a life-threatening dysrhythmia, also giving the person an inappropriate shock. This itself can stimulate a life-threatening dysrhythmia. Because of this, those with AICDs should be closely monitored during exercise. The upper limit for target heart rate with exercise should be set at least 10 bpm below the programmed heart rate at which point the device would deliver a shock.[2]

Chapter 4

Stress and Other Risk Factors

The American Heart Association and The American College of Sports Medicine identify seven primary risk factors for heart disease. Whether or not you currently suffer from heart disease, chances are good that you possess at least one risk factor. Some risk factors are modifiable, meaning we can improve on them by making lifestyle changes. The modifiable risk factors include:

- Cigarette smoking
- Hypertension (high blood pressure)
- Dyslipidemia (high cholesterol)
- Impaired fasting blood glucose (high blood sugar)
- Obesity
- Sedentary lifestyle
- Stress

Other concerns are non-modifiable, meaning no matter what we do, we have no control over them. Here are risk factors in that category:

- Family history
- Age
- Gender

For example, in terms of family history, if you are a man and have a parent with an early heart attack, your risk for having a heart attack doubles. If you are a female with a similar history, your risk increases by about 70%.[1]

The information in this chapter can be useful to you in determining how great your risk is for heart disease, or can simply guide you toward identifying aspects of your health that need improvement.

These modifiable or non-modifiable risk factors can further be divided into primary and secondary risk factors. Primary risk factors are those with a strong link to heart disease. Secondary risk factors can also lead to heart disease, but as independent risk factors, the association is not as strong.[2]

Family History
This is a primary non-modifiable risk factor where a father or other male first-

degree relative (e.g. brother) suffers from a myocardial infarction, coronary revascularization (CABG, PTCA, etc.) or sudden death before age 55, or a mother or female first-degree relative (e.g. sister) before age 65. Your chances of heart disease increase if you meet these criteria.

Knowing that family history is one of my risk factors for heart disease, I need to be especially mindful of my current lifestyle habits. You see, my father had a heart attack at 42 years of age. It started when he was at home complaining of jaw pain. The pain gradually intensified on that Saturday morning to the point where my mother drove him to a walk-in medical center. There it was determined he was indeed having a heart attack. He ended up having an angioplasty.

My father had learned the hard way of the significance of family history for heart disease. My grandfather had his heart attack at age 59. And although by definition this may not qualify since he was older than 55 at the time, all three of my grandfather's sisters had coronary artery disease. It is safe to assume heart disease is prevalent in my family.

My father was initially doing well after his procedure. He exercised on an Airdyne bike in our basement, utilizing both upper and lower extremities for aerobics. He would also frequently go on brisk walks for 30 to 60 minutes, and he took his medications.

Unfortunately, this compliance did not last with his exercise regimen. It was also easy for him to gain weight, which placed additional strain on his heart. When his cardiologist retired, my father didn't see the need to find another one. He assumed his annual check-up appointments with his primary care physician were enough.

However, at age 59, my father failed a stress test, which led to the discovery of a major blockage in his coronary arteries. This should not have been a surprise since he revealed that he had been feeling fatigued, not motivated to do much, and depressed for quite some time, symptoms he unfortunately did not think to mention to his physician right away. He ended up having quadruple bypass surgery at age 59, the same age his father had his heart event!

Now my father has a cardiologist whom he sees twice a year for a checkup. He also sees his primary care physician twice a year for a physical. He now feels confident that all of his health issues are addressed by seeing one of these two doctors every three months. Due to his cardiac history, it is comforting to my father and to his family that he is under the care of a specialist who is focused on his cardiovascular health.

Age

This is a secondary risk factor which, like family history, is non-modifiable. What this means is the older we get, the more at risk we are for heart disease. This is why the American College of Sports Medicine (ACSM) recommends a stress test prior to vigorous exercise for men over 45 and women over 55 years of age.[3] Just as there is wear and tear on an older car with high mileage, the coronary arteries tend to harden, with a greater buildup of plaque as we age, leading to a greater risk of a heart attack. Although the impact of a heart attack remains greater in men compared to women, the gender difference tends to narrow as men and women continue to age.[4] In other words, the older we get, the more the risk of a heart attack is nearly equal among men and women.

In my experience in the surgical ICU, the average age I see with CABG or valve repair is around 65 years old. It's not uncommon for me to see patients in their late 70s recovering from those surgical procedures as well. Although I have seen patients in their 80s with the surgery, this is not too common. The recovery period tends to be much more complicated. The ones I have seen who were older and had a successful outcome tended to be in good shape prior to the procedure. This is a characteristic I've observed in younger patients as well. What I hope you take from this message is that as you age, the importance of regular exercise and a heart-healthy diet cannot be emphasized enough.

Gender

Another risk factor that needs to be considered is whether or not your gender is putting you at greater risk for a heart attack because of certain social behavior patterns that are gender specific. For example, when it comes to heart disease, women tend to be underdiagnosed. Statistics show that younger males are more prone to heart attacks than females, especially young females, which may give younger females a false sense of security about their own risks for a heart attack. Furthermore, women are less likely to experience "classical" symptoms such as chest pain or shortness of breath, which may explain why they are reluctant to seek swift medical attention.

A patient I worked with for several months, Jane, did experience the classical symptoms, and, when it was revealed that she had a blockage in her coronary artery, many people were surprised to hear that such a young woman had that condition. As Jane explains in her interview, shared at greater length toward the end of the next chapter, "Cardiovascular Training: Frequency and Duration," she felt "scared and ashamed," as if having a blockage was her fault. This is not uncommon when faced with a disease that statistics show you're not supposed to get.

Therefore, if you are a woman, you need to work on the mindset, if you have it, that men more often have to worry about getting a heart attack and look at yourself and your own risk factors very carefully. Several "unclassical" symptoms women should be aware of are fatigue, nausea, and GI symptoms mimicking acid reflux, such as heartburn.

If you are a man, be careful that you are not falling into the traps that too many men do, especially an avoidance of regular physical checkups with the accompanying blood work that might confirm whether or not you have developed any or several of the risk factors for heart disease since your last checkup. Pay attention especially to whether or not you have high blood pressure, high cholesterol, and high blood sugar, all treatable conditions with medication, as well as the lifestyle risk factors of obesity, cigarette smoking, or sedentary lifestyle.

Cigarette Smoking
If you are a current smoker or have quit within the previous six months, you are at an increased risk for heart disease. This modifiable risk factor limits the number of oxygen-rich blood cells that travel to the heart. Besides the greater risk of heart disease, exercise tolerance can be significantly reduced. This should be of little surprise, since less oxygen-rich blood cells will reach our body's tissues. This may explain why you may have noticed smokers engaging in physical activity tend to huff and puff a little more often than their non-smoking counterparts.

Unlike family history, cigarette smoking is a modifiable risk factor. Because of the increased odds of having a heart attack due to smoking, it is in your best interest to quit.

There are a variety of methods and treatments available for smoking cessation that have been used successfully by smokers who want to quit, even the heaviest of "chain" smokers. Some individuals have successfully quit "cold turkey." They simply decided to stop smoking and have refrained from picking up another cigarette. As encouraging as this may sound, however, few manage to quit so effortlessly. Recidivism is high among former smokers, especially when others in the household or more than a few friends continue to smoke. Other smokers looking to quit may require more aggressive therapy, possibly by participating in a support group, with or without the addition of pharmacological treatment. A combination of drugs and behavioral change seem to make the greatest impact.

One option is a nicotine patch (e.g. Nicoderm˙). This is a patch that should be applied above the waist and below the neck to an area of clean, dry, hairless skin. It provides a measured dose of nicotine and can be purchased without a prescription. Doses are tapered down over a course of several weeks. The Food and Drug Administration (FDA) recommends using this product for no longer than five months.

Nicotine gum (e.g. Nicorette˙) is a fast-acting form of nicotine absorbed through the mouth. This is also purchased without a prescription. The recommended duration of usage is one to three months; and no longer than six months. The major drawback is that people often become dependent on this gum. It is not uncommon to find people chewing this product more than a year after quitting smoking.

Nicotine lozenges are another oral form of administration, also available without a prescription. They are used for 12 weeks, tapering down the dosage throughout the duration.

A nicotine nasal spray (e.g. Nicotrol NS˙) is one option that provides immediate relief of withdrawal symptoms. The FDA recommends using this product for no longer than six months. This product is available only with a prescription.

A nicotine inhaler (also by Nicotrol˙) is another fast-acting form of nicotine administration. Nicotine inhalers deliver most of the nicotine vapor into the mouth, whereas most other inhalers deliver to the lungs. This is also available only with a prescription.

Chantix˙ is a prescription drug called a nicotine receptor agonist. It helps decrease withdrawal symptoms and curbs nicotine cravings. Treatment should begin one week prior to quitting smoking, since it takes about a week for the medicine to take effect. It should be used for a 12-week period, and should not be used in conjunction with any other smoking cessation product. This medicine should especially not be used along with a nicotine patch unless directed by your doctor, due to an increase in blood pressure. If the desired effect is not achieved in the 12-week period, Chantix˙ can be taken for an additional 12 weeks.

Wellbutrin˙ and Zyban˙ are medicines used to treat depression, with an added benefit of helping people quit smoking. They do this by blocking the flow of chemicals in the brain responsible for the intense craving. Similar to Chantix,˙ these medicines should be initiated one week prior to quitting and should be used for seven to 12 weeks.[5] If you already take medicine for depression, a different medication should be used to help quit smoking. It should also not be used in conjunction with the nicotine patch for that same increase in blood pressure, unless directed by your doctor.[5]

If you feel you need additional support, there are many resources available to you. Look for smoking cessation programs in your local hospitals, or through the local branch of the American Cancer Society or the American Lung Association. There are also support groups such as Smokers Anonymous, as well as hotlines with trained staff.

There are many other unconventional methods of quitting that have helped a number of people, including acupuncture, hypnosis, switching from drinking coffee to tea, and abstaining from alcohol. It's important to identify your personal triggers to smoking and work on eliminating them. Ultimately, it will take trial and error to determine which methods of quitting will work best for you.

One of the greatest barriers to quitting smoking among those I've worked with is when others in their household continue to smoke. You could have the best intentions of quitting, but when a spouse or other loved one continues to smoke, the familiar temptations begin to intensify.

Those successful in quitting began by setting ground rules (e.g. no smoking in the house, etc.). If your loved ones are truly supportive, they will make the necessary adjustments. It might even encourage them to kick the habit as well. Regardless of their actions, you must be strong enough to take responsibility for your own actions. After all, yours are the ones you ultimately control.

If you slip and have a cigarette after quitting, accept the fact that it was just a slip. You don't necessarily have to label yourself as a smoker, finish the pack, and search for more. Instead, think about what caused you to reach for that cigarette in the first place and what you could do differently in the future to resist this temptation. Ultimately, *you* are the one in control. Make the decision to just throw the pack away and start fresh!

Hypertension

This modifiable risk factor can be defined as having a systolic blood pressure (top number) of <u>over</u> 140mmHg or a diastolic blood pressure (bottom number) of <u>over</u> 90mmHg. This would need to be confirmed by measurement on at least two separate occasions. Other criteria would be if you're currently taking antihypertensive medications.

Two different stages of hypertension exist, representing severity of the illness. Stage I hypertension can be defined as a systolic blood pressure of 140-159mmHg or a diastolic blood pressure of 90-99mmHg. Stage II hypertension represents a systolic blood pressure of 160mmHg or <u>over</u> or a diastolic blood pressure 100mmHg or <u>over</u>.

Prehypertension is a term used to classify those with a systolic blood pressure of 120-139mmHg or a diastolic blood pressure of 84-89mmHg. Although not a risk factor, it does indicate those at risk for developing hypertension in the future. You can think of it as a warning sign. Although antihypertensive medications are not usually prescribed for prehypertension, it would indicate the need for dietary and exercise interventions. Normal blood pressure formerly was considered 120/80mmHg. Current guidelines have become stricter, indicating 115/75mmHg as the desirable levels. The importance of successful blood pressure management is not only to reduce the risk for heart disease, but also to reduce the risk for stroke and kidney disease. Become familiar with where your blood pressure normally runs. Schedule routine physicals to ensure your blood pressure is appropriately managed and well-controlled.

Dyslipidemia

This modifiable risk factor can be defined as an LDL (bad cholesterol) <u>over</u> 130mg/dL or HDL (good cholesterol) of <u>under</u> 40mg/dL. Milligrams per deciliter (mg/dL) is the unit of measurement to determine the amount of a substance in the blood, whether it be cholesterol or glucose, etc. If the only available information on the blood panel is total cholesterol, a value of more than 200mg/dL would be a risk factor. For those already suffering from heart disease, the guidelines have become stricter, where LDL should be <u>under</u> 100mg/dL. For those with congestive heart failure (CHF) and more complicated types of heart disease, cardiologists are looking for LDL <u>under</u> 70mg/dL and total cholesterol <u>under</u> 180mg/dL. With regards to total cholesterol and LDL, the lower the value the better.

Dietary control is a necessity for those with this risk factor. Unfortunately, it could be a problem with genetics whereby, regardless of the type of diet you follow, you could still have abnormal values. If diet and exercise are insufficient in managing your cholesterol level, medications may need to be added. (See Chapter 12 for a discussion of cholesterol-lowering medications).

Impaired Fasting Blood Glucose

This risk factor is defined as having a fasting blood glucose reading of <u>over</u> 100 mg/dL, confirmed by measurement on at least two separate occasions. With a high glucose level in the blood, the heart has to pump this sticky blood through the walls of the arteries. This can exacerbate the risk of clogging the arteries, leading to significant blockages, heart attack, stroke, etc. Adults being treated for diabetes are just as likely to have a heart attack or stroke or die from cardiovascular causes as those with a prior heart attack. They're also twice as likely as non-diabetics to die after a heart attack. I consider this a modifiable risk factor because with proper diet, exercise, and possibly certain medications, you can exert some control over this value. Glucose-lowering medications will be covered in a later chapter.

Obesity

This modifiable risk factor is recognized as having a body mass index (BMI) of over 30 kg/m² or a waist girth of over 102 cm for males and over 88 cm for females, or a waist/hip ratio of over 0.95 for males and over 0.86 for females. BMI uses your body weight in kilograms divided by your height in meters squared. Square meters refers to the total area an object takes up. People should be cautious when using BMI to identify obesity. Because muscle weighs more than fat, a very muscular individual can be mislabeled as obese or even morbidly obese, yet have a normal waist circumference and normal waist/hip ratio.

Take myself, for example. I am five feet seven inches tall and weigh 240 pounds. According to my BMI, I am considered obese. My ideal body weight based on a height and weight chart is around 165 pounds. However, because of the amount of muscle mass I am carrying, it would not be suitable for me to drop so much weight, considering my body fat percentage is at a healthy 10%. Despite the 70-pound "excess" weight, my blood pressure, cholesterol and overall endurance are more than adequate. The point is, it would be wise *not* to use BMI independently. Including waist circumference and/or waist/hip ratio along with BMI would provide greater accuracy, considering those carrying a greater percentage of fat stored in the abdomen are at a heightened health risk.

I have worked with numerous obese clients in the past 11 years, as well as several morbidly obese individuals. Depending upon how many other risk factors they presented, exercise was uniquely structured to each individual. Each one's overall success was determined by how consistent they were with their diet and exercise program.

A common question I am asked is whether obese individuals can safely and efficiently begin an exercise program or should focus on losing the weight first. This question usually baffles me because I cannot see how they would lose the weight without following an exercise program. Sure, we can all lose weight if we starve ourselves. But what is going to encourage your body to use stored fat as its energy source, thus burning fat? Exercise!

Although exercise can be safe and effective for obese individuals, modifications often need to be made. For starters, obese individuals do not usually have great stamina, especially if they are new to exercise. As a result, it may not be realistic for them to complete 40 to 60 minutes of aerobic activity in one shot. Short, intermittent sessions of 10 to 20 minutes may initially be more suitable.

If using machines for aerobics, it may be difficult to find a suitable one. The average treadmill has a 300- to 400-pound maximum weight limit. Contact the manufacturer or refer to the manual of the specific treadmill to determine weight capacity. Seated machines such as recumbent bikes need to be wide enough so the individual can get in and out with relative ease. I am happy to see that newer machines tend to be catered to the larger individual; having wider seats, greater space and higher weight capacities.

Resistance training should be included in the obese individual's regimen to help speed up metabolism and encourage weight loss. Initially, machines should be emphasized to encourage proper lifting technique. If machines are not available, doing exercises with your body weight can be effective, such as chair squats or a squat on the wall with a Swiss ball (Refer to Chapter 7 for descriptions of these exercises). With regard to Swiss balls, the average 65-cm Swiss ball has a weight capacity of 600 pounds! Most obese individuals need not worry. Although they may have some physical limitations, there are clearly a great number of aerobic and resistance exercise options for them to add to a low-calorie diet for the best possible results.

The greatest amount of weight loss that I have seen in a client of mine is about 60 pounds. This loss was over a six-month period. Unfortunately, I don't have the opportunity to see such dramatic changes in all of my clients. Part of the reason is they usually start cardiac rehab shortly after their heart event and are with me for only three months (if they are good with attendance). Such changes usually take longer to achieve. The upcoming chapters on exercise and nutrition should help with you or your loved one's weight loss goals if obesity is one of your modifiable risk factors.

Sedentary Lifestyle

This primary modifiable risk factor is caused by being physically inactive. The more technical criteria is if someone is not participating in a regular exercise program or meeting the minimal physical activity recommendations from the U.S. Surgeon General's Report, which recommends engaging in greater than 30 minutes of moderate physical activity on most days of the week.[6]

Those spending numerous hours per day behind a desk or in front of a television set during the day or at night and on weekends make up a large percentage of the population exhibiting this risk factor. In fact, a recent study cosponsored by the National Cancer Institute and the American Association of Retired Persons (AARP) showed that people with higher levels of sedentary behaviors (i.e. prolonged TV watching, computer work, etc.) had higher mortality rates compared with more active individuals. This is true even when participating in the minimum recommended levels of moderate physical activity.[7]

Negative Risk Factor for Heart Disease

There is actually one more primary risk factor that is unique and recognized as a negative risk factor for heart disease: having an HDL (good cholesterol) level of over 60 mg/dL. A negative risk factor simply means that if you have additional risk factors along with a negative risk factor, you can eliminate one of your other risk factors. So if you had three positive risk factors and also had this negative risk factor, you would really have just two positive risk factors. If you recall, I mentioned that with total cholesterol and LDL, the lower the value the better. Regarding HDL, a higher value is most desirable. I consider this a modifiable risk factor, because with lifestyle changes such as resistance training and omega-3 fatty acid consumption, we can improve our HDL value. Although we may not be able to achieve an HDL of over 60 mg/dL, we can surely improve our current value. I've personally seen great improvements in HDL cholesterol by implementing some of these exercise and dietary changes to know that positive benefits can be achieved. Any improvement, no matter how small, can be significant.

To this point, I've identified the primary risk factors for heart disease. There are additional risk factors and, although they don't have as strong a link to heart disease, they can still pose a threat. I will address modifiable and non-modifiable secondary risk factors. Take notice how much more attention I devote to the modifiable risk factors, since many interventions exist for a substantial reduction.

Depression

Over the past 15 years, a link has been identified between depression and heart disease. Clinically depressed individuals are at a significantly greater risk of a heart attack, even after controlling for primary risk factors such as hypertension, smoking, obesity, physical inactivity and family history.[8] Studies show even mild depression is associated with an increased risk for acute coronary syndrome and all-cause mortality in patients with established heart disease.[9]

But this secondary risk factor can be considered modifiable since effective treatments do exist. Unfortunately, depression often goes undiagnosed and therefore goes untreated. One explanation is that doctors and cardiologists may misinterpret signs and symptoms of depression for medication adjustments or secondary side effects due to patients recovering from their cardiac event.

Fortunately, there are tests and screening processes available to help determine if you are clinically depressed. One such screening was published by the National Institute of Mental Health (NIMH) in 2002.[10] If you suffer from five or more of the following symptoms for at least two weeks and that interferes with work, self-care, child-care and/or social activities, you should contact your physician:

1. Persistent sad, anxious or "empty" mood
2. Feelings of hopelessness or pessimism
3. Feelings of guilt, worthlessness or helplessness
4. Loss of interest or pleasure in hobbies and activities once enjoyed, including sex
5. Decreased energy; fatigue
6. Difficulty concentrating, remembering, decision-making
7. Insomnia, early-morning awakening, or oversleeping
8. Changes in appetite and/or weight
9. Thoughts of death, suicide or suicide attempts
10. Restlessness, irritability

Although the exact cause of depression is not known, a couple of treatments exist with good success: *medication* and a form of psychotherapy called *cognitive behavioral therapy* (CBT). The medication of choice is selective serotonin reuptake inhibitors (SSRI). Examples include Lexapro˚ and Paxil˚. CBT focuses on the current symptoms, thoughts and behaviors of the patient. The American Institute for Cognitive Therapy in New York City claims that with 20 sessions of individual therapy, approximately 75% of patients experience a significant decrease in their symptoms. With medication added, the efficacy increases to 85%!

I've worked with several clients who were depressed. Some discovered exercise alone was enough for full recovery. Others required additional treatment with a therapist. If you feel you may suffer from depression, don't hesitate to contact your physician. If depression is left untreated, the evidence indicates your risk for a future heart event only escalates.

Stress

Psychological stress is present in all of our lives. It may be positive stress, such as getting married, having a baby, getting a great job or a postgraduate degree, or planning a big party. These positive stresses are known as *eustress.*

Or it can be negative stress, such as problems at work, unemployment, financial worries or marital problems. These negative stresses are known as *distress.*

Whether the stress is positive or negative, too much of it over a prolonged period could result in serious health problems. Although stress may not be recognized as a major risk factor for heart disease, it is accepted in the medical community as playing a role in the progression of heart disease.

If we think of the physical symptoms of acute stress, it is no mystery how stress can be a risk factor for heart disease. With acute stress comes the activation of the autonomic nervous system, which increases our heart rate and blood pressure. Prolonged stress may impair our immune system, which can increase our susceptibility to illness. High levels of stress may negatively influence health behaviors such as smoking, diet, exercise, and use of medications.[11]

Symptoms of stress are often similar to symptoms of depression and anxiety. Examples include difficulty sleeping, fatigue, muscle tension and soreness, changes in appetite, headaches, and gastrointestinal problems. High levels of stress can place individuals at risk for more serious mental or physical health problems. Therefore, it is important to develop coping skills enabling us to gain better control of the problems in our lives. When we talk about stress, we are talking about feeling a loss of control.

Interventions for stress exist, helping us feel in control and developing problem-focused coping skills. Examples include our social support networks, family and friends, self-help groups, and religious services. Exercise can be another great stress-reliever. When we exercise, there is a release of hormones called endorphins, which promote feelings of well-being. Exercise helps release built-up tension in our bodies, as well as providing a venue for releasing emotional tension. Exercise can also raise feelings of self-esteem. Some forms of exercise allow you to be social, which can also be great for stress reduction.

One other intervention to reduce stress is guided imagery. Guided imagery is a kind of directed, deliberate daydream; a purposeful creation of positive sensory images (sight, sound, taste, smell, and feel) in our imagination. It has been shown to be a way of using the imagination very specifically to help the mind and body heal, stay strong, and even perform as needed.[12]

Benefits of imagery include combating fear, isolation, illness, depression, and anxiety.[12] It helps provide hope, optimism and peace of mind. It has been helpful with illnesses like cancer, stroke, heart disease, multiple sclerosis, rheumatoid arthritis, diabetes and HIV, and situations like surgeries and chemotherapy. New studies are showing benefits in combating post-traumatic stress disorder (PTSD) and panic attacks. Dr. Jennifer Strauss, a principal investigator at Duke University Medical Center and Durham V.A. Hospital, has shown in her randomized, placebo-controlled pilot study the positive impact guided imagery has in those suffering from PTSD.[13] A study published in 2007 showed the benefits of diet modification, exercise, and mind-body stress reduction methods to reduce the coronary risk in both men and women.[14]

Guided imagery has also been helpful with self-confidence, especially with athletes. When asked about their high shooting percentages, basketball players often remark about envisioning the hoop like a large hula hoop, while the basketball is no larger than a softball. With this "imagery," they feel it's impossible for that ball not to sink.

I've shared similar success with imagery in my own sport. Prior to a bodybuilding competition, while pumping up minutes before going out on stage, watching the numerous nationally ranked competitors in phenomenal shape can really psych you out and wreak havoc on your confidence. This can be even more pronounced in a depleted and dehydrated state, which is the norm at this point. You feel too skinny and small in comparison to these "extra-large beasts." This low self-confidence can easily be reflected on stage in front of the judges and can leave you beating yourself before the contest even begins! By listening to a particular guided imagery CD entitled, "Self-Confidence" daily for two weeks prior to contest time, I was backstage feeling like an "extra-large beast" myself; one that would not go down without a fight! For the last couple of weeks before every contest, I make sure I listen to that CD daily for that competitive edge. So far, it hasn't let me down.

In her book *Staying Well with Guided Imagery*, psychotherapist Belleruth Naparstek identified three principles of imagery:[12]

1. *Our bodies don't discriminate between what is real and sensory images of the mind.* In other words, our bodies don't know the difference from what is real or imaginary.

2. *In the altered state, we are capable of more rapid and intense healing, growth, learning and change.* Basically, we are more receptive to change when in the altered state; this complete relaxation and temporary dissociation from reality.

3. *We feel better about ourselves when we have a sense of mastery over what is happening to us.* One common characteristic of people who are under considerable stress is having the feeling of loss of control. This third principle is saying that by feeling we have control over the challenging situations in our lives, we'll feel better about ourselves.

Putting these principles together, if we introduce images to the mind that the body believes are actual events, and doing this in the altered state; doing it when, how and where we want to, we have at our command the unique, powerful and versatile technique of guided imagery.

Guided imagery can utilize many mind-body tools, such as relaxing your muscles with a full-body scan. It can include relaxing music. It often includes focusing on your breathing. I remember hearing Belleruth Naparstek at a conference in Danbury, Connecticut, in 2007. She told a story of how she helped a witness to the tragedy in New York City on September 11, 2001. When the Twin Towers fell, one of the many eyewitnesses to this event was panicking and running hysterically. She couldn't seem to pull herself together. Belleruth went up to this hysterical woman, placed her hands on the woman's shoulders and asked her to just look in her eyes and breathe with her. Belleruth had her inhale, counting "1, 2, 3," and exhaling, counting "1, 2, 3." This continued for several minutes.

Before long, the panicking woman was calmed down and had regained self-control in this chaotic environment. This is an example of the power of these mind-body tools. By focusing on her body, she was able to dissociate from what was happening all around her.

Another useful tool that can enhance imagery is touch. With touch, we have the ability to make images more vivid, intense and emotionally present than they might otherwise be. It is especially beneficial for those with respiratory problems, such as chronic obstructive pulmonary disease, where focusing on breathing might not be such a relaxing experience. An example of imagery with touch would be when you place your hands on your abdomen, as an anchoring device. You feel your belly as you breathe in and out. After practicing this for several sessions, the simple act of placing your hands on your belly should be enough of a cue to get you into that state of relaxation.

Psychotherapists have found that repetitive listening to guided imagery tapes seemed to intensify and speed up the work of therapy. Simply put, practice makes perfect. The more you use it, the more your response to it deepens, intensifies, and becomes more controllable.

For those who wish to practice guided imagery, you can start by finding a nice quiet area, closing your eyes, and paying attention to your breathing. As Belleruth did with the woman in New York City, you can focus on counting to three as you inhale, and again as you exhale. You can include playing a tape of relaxing music or even a guided imagery tape. Belleruth sells a variety of tapes and compact discs focusing on various topics, illnesses and ailments (cardiovascular disease, COPD, cancer, preparing for surgery, low self-esteem, etc.). You can view her collection at http://www.healthjourneys.com. You can even create your own tape of your own soothing voice, perhaps with some relaxing background music to enhance the experience.

The remainder of this chapter will share my writings of a full-body scan, which include some guided imagery I use in my own practice. Feel free to copy this onto a tape with your own voice or make whatever modifications you find necessary. During this exercise, it's not a problem if your mind wanders and isn't totally focused on my words. Just accept what comes into your mind. The clearest, truest images show up when we take a receptive attitude and just allow images to come in as if they had a life of their own. Believe it or not, they do have a life of their own. Ultimately, you are in control. Any thoughts or images you feel are unnecessary and serve no purpose, simply allow them to fade away as easily as they enter your mind.

Guided Imagery – Body Scan

Begin by sitting comfortably with your eyes closed, feet flat on the floor, with your back against the chair. Try to keep your head, neck, and spine as straight as you can, as you take a deep cleansing breath in…(pause)… and slowly let it out … and again … take a deep breath in … (pause)… and slowly let it out … (pause).

As you continue to breathe each cleansing breath in, allow your lungs and all of your body's tissues to fill with the fresh, clean, oxygen-rich air … (pause) … and with each breath out … allowing all wastes, toxins and negative energy to slowly be released … leaving your body feeling more and more relaxed … (pause) … any negative thoughts, worries, and emotions fading away, as they are not needed at this time. Try for a few moments to just focus on you and your body. At this time, allow your muscles to relax by participating in a full-body scan.

Begin by bringing your attention to your feet and toes … ankles and shins … (pause) … allowing these areas of your body to just hang loose …

feeling free of any tension, tightness, soreness, or discomfort ... (pause). Allow the oxygen-rich blood to flow to these areas at this time ... (pause)... moving up now to your thighs and hips ... buttocks and pelvic region ... (pause)... Allow these muscles to relax in the chair, releasing any tension or discomfort that may be present ... (pause). Make yourself aware of the feeling of the coldness or warmth of the chair you're sitting on ... (pause). Move on now to the muscles of your lower back, middle back, and upper back ... (pause)... allowing these muscles to loosen and relax against the back of the chair... allowing the chair to do all of the work in supporting your body upright ... (pause).

Move now to your chest muscle ... working down to your abdomen ... (pause) ... Try to relax your stomach ... soften your belly...allowing free and easy breathing ... (pause)... any worries or fears that may be present in your belly, allow it to work its way out as you exhale completely ... (pause). Moving now to the muscles of your shoulders ... arms ... forearms ... hands ... and fingers ... (pause)... your index fingers ... middle fingers ... ring fingers... pinkies ... and thumbs ... (pause)... Allow these areas of your body to just hang loose, letting go of any built-up tension, tightness, or discomfort ... (pause).

Now try focusing on your forehead ... cheeks ... jaw ... allowing the jaw to just hang loose, as you soften all of your facial muscles ... including the muscles surrounding your eyes ... (pause)... Now bring your attention to your neck. The neck is an area of your body that tends to tighten when under stress, leaving a feeling like a huge knot has been tied. To take full advantage of this relaxation period, as you breathe this next breath in ... allow that knot to loosen ... (pause). As you let go of that breath ... that knot totally becomes untied, leaving you with a new sense of freedom ... Feeling like a huge weight has been lifted off of your shoulders... (pause).

At this time, your body should feel as light as feather, floating in midair. Enjoy this feeling ... remember it. Keep in mind that anytime you wish to return here, you can easily do so by simply finding a nice quiet area ... paying attention to your breathing ... and focusing on relaxing the various muscles of your body.

As this session now comes to a close, you can end with one last deep breath in ... and as you let that breath out ... you can bring your attention back into the room ... (pause). When you feel ready, you can begin to slowly open your eyes ... and enjoy the rest of your day... knowing you are better for it.

Keep in mind that although relaxation techniques, such as guided imagery and meditation, are very effective for a variety of conditions, there are situations where they are not enough. In the case of severe depression or anxiety, for example, psychotherapy and/or medication may also be needed. Do not hesitate to contact your doctor if you are suffering from symptoms such as persistent feelings of sadness or irritability, feelings of guilt, worthlessness or helplessness, sleep disturbances, change in appetite, loss of interest in previously enjoyed activities, difficulty thinking or concentrating, or thoughts of death or suicide.

Reflecting on all of these risk factors I've discussed, a connection can be made among many of the modifiable risk factors. Although we can't do anything to change our family history, nor can we go back in time and be five years old again, we can certainly modify these other risk factors. Like a row of dominos, if you knock one down, the rest will soon follow. Make exercise your first domino. By getting an exercise regimen started, you will burn calories, which will help you lose weight. Furthermore, you will tend to eat healthier to give yourself fuel for a better workout. You will probably end up quitting smoking because you'll find breathing a heck of a lot easier when exercising after quitting. If you have diabetes, you will most likely experience improved glucose readings, related to exercise and proper nutrition. You should also expect to see improvements in both blood pressure and cholesterol, related to exercise and proper diet. Lastly, exercise will release certain hormones and other chemicals in the blood such as serotonin, norepinephrine, endorphins and GABA, which will help reduce stress, anxiety, depression, heart rate, blood pressure, and muscle tension. As you can see, one small positive change can lead to an array of positive changes.

Part 2

Exercise

Chapter 5

Why Exercise, and What's Stopping You?

Elizabeth is a 76-year-old grandmother who has been an active participant in a phase III non-monitored cardiac rehab exercise program for the past seven years. Here is her story:

I think it would not be an overstatement to say that in my 76 years, I have gathered a "little bit" of life experience. I have always had to work hard to make a living, but that was never much of a problem because I had the energy and health (or so I thought) to do it. If I saw someone get sick or suffer a tragedy, I surely empathized with them, but also felt like "that could never happen to me." As such, I did not pay attention to my health.

It bothered me that I was continuously gaining weight, but not enough to do anything about it. In addition to obesity, I had high blood pressure and type II diabetes. My doctors warned me countless times to exercise or at least find time to take daily walks, since I sat behind a desk for 10 to 12 hours a day working as an accountant. I ignored them. I continued to do my stressful work and live life in a completely sedentary way. I paid no attention to my diet whatsoever. This continued until winter of 2003.

Then, in late December, I had seen my cardiologist for a routine physical and passed with flying colors. Why did I see a cardiologist, you may ask? Upon arriving in the U.S. from Hungary over 20 years ago, I knew I needed to find a good primary care physician. With a family history of heart problems, I felt it would be best to have a heart specialist as my general practitioner.

Two weeks after this appointment, I went back to see my doctor, for I was feeling unusually tired and short of breath. I wasn't thinking "heart" when I saw him on January 3rd. At the time, it was a struggle to walk from one end of the room to the other.

After listening to my lungs, he ordered a stat chest x-ray, for he did not like what he'd heard. Upon obtaining the results, he sent me to the emergency department at the nearest hospital due to fluid on my lungs. It was also evident that there were changes on my EKG compared to my physical two weeks prior. It was found that I had three blockages in my coronary arteries, resulting in triple bypass surgery, along with mitral valve repair.

To make matters worse, I had several complications post-operatively. I developed congestive heart failure, which caused more fluid on my lungs as my heart was unable to pump blood as well as it should. A biventricular pacemaker was inserted to give my heart the "help" it needed. My blood pressure was apparently dropping and I wasn't getting adequate perfusion to my kidneys, which landed me in kidney failure and on dialysis.

During my two-and-a-half-month stay in the hospital, I believe I had three or four dialysis treatments, which was not a fun experience. A typical session would leave me feeling completely exhausted for the rest of the day. I felt good for nothing!

Most of my time in the hospital was spent in the ICU, which thankfully was mostly a blur. It was difficult to get me off of the breathing machine, which I now believe had to do with my obesity and sedentary lifestyle.

Before leaving ICU, the nurses had moved me from my all-too-familiar bed to a recliner chair. It amazed me how simply sliding from the bed to the chair wiped me out so much. Due to my length of stay in ICU, by the time I was moving to the recliner chair, my chest incision was healing well enough where the pain was not too bad. It was the fatigue that was most troubling.

Before being discharged from the hospital, I had spent three weeks on a rehab unit. This was not a pleasurable experience. The nurses and physical therapists had insisted I get out of the bed and chair and start walking. I remember my first time out of bed. I could barely walk a few steps without feeling completely winded. I felt like I just couldn't do it.

The turning point for me was when I glanced out in the hallway and noticed patients successfully walking up and down the hallway. I saw others out in the hall scurrying around, attending to their business. This upset me a great deal because I felt so helpless. I did some soul-searching and told myself that I would not allow myself to be dependent on others and be wheelchair-bound. I needed to stop feeling sorry for myself and get moving! Although it was very difficult, I worked at it with the help of the staff and after three weeks of rehab, I walked out of the hospital on my own two feet.

The same inner strength I found in the hospital, I channeled towards a new task: increasing my physical strength and cardiovascular endurance in a cardiac rehab program. It was scary at first, with the staff making me walk on treadmills and pedaling on bikes. I must admit I was worried my heart wouldn't be able to take it. Here again, I felt weak and tired with little activity, especially compared to many of the other participants.

Initially, I was discouraged and constantly looked for reasons why I couldn't attend. I was stubborn, though, and not willing to return to my old sedentary ways. My husband was not well, himself. He was battling with stomach cancer. He needed a wife who could do for herself, so she'd be able to care for his needs as well. You could say I had a lot of motivation to get myself in better shape.

Upon completion of the program, I was not only able to handle all of the exercises, I was able to do them continuously for forty minutes! I even learned how to incorporate weight training in my exercise routine. What has been particularly rewarding has been how the exercise in cardiac rehab has enhanced my ability to do household chores and leisure activities. It has even worked wonders in my posture and balance. It is especially rewarding for me to be able to play and keep up with my five-year-old granddaughter, who is a ball of energy! I could not imagine taking her to the park and swinging her on the swing how I was six years ago.

Although I have made great improvements, I accept the fact that I need to keep up with exercise and healthy behaviors for the rest of my life. During recent months, I had lost my husband who became very ill. Not only am I grateful for the good-quality years together, I am grateful that my health was good enough to be there and take care of him during his final days.

Even though he is gone, it is not acceptable for me to feel sorry for myself. I still have much to live for, including a son, daughter-in-law, and beautiful granddaughter who needs her grandma. Because of my devotion to exercise, I believe I will continue to enjoy many good-quality years with them.

Our lives are gifts, and we only get one chance to make the most of them. We are each responsible for our own well-being. No one can force us to eat a healthy diet, exercise, or make the right choices. It is up to each individual. Exercise requires continuous discipline and dedication, and I am living proof that it is as important to life as food and water. Start today – and don't stop!

Benefits of Exercise

As Elizabeth's story demonstrates, there are health benefits linked with regular exercise such as a reduction in the resting heart rate and blood pressure, increased HDL (good) cholesterol and decreased LDL (bad) cholesterol, reduced total body fat, reduced blood platelet adhesiveness and aggregation (sticky blood), improved glucose tolerance (decreased insulin requirements), decreasing of the workload on the heart, and increased bone density (stronger bones).

There is also a strong correlation with exercise to decreased anxiety and depression, enhanced feelings of well-being, and a better ability to perform work, recreational and sports activities. This all equates to better physical functioning and independent living in older adults.[1]

Physical inactivity has been identified as a primary risk factor for heart disease, along with many other associated medical conditions, such as obesity, type II diabetes mellitus and osteoporosis, to name a few. Just what is the physical activity I'm referring to? It can be defined as bodily movement produced by the contraction of our skeletal muscles that increases our energy expenditure.

Exercise is just one type of physical activity, which is a planned, structured and repetitive body movement done to improve or maintain one or more components of physical fitness.[1]

Physical fitness is a very broad term, which can be broken up into several components. There are skill-related components, which include speed, power, agility, balance, and coordination. There are health-related aspects, which include muscular strength and endurance, cardiovascular endurance, flexibility, and body composition. There is also a physiologic component to fitness, which includes our metabolism, such as how well our bodies can transport glucose into our cells, which is a problem for those with diabetes. Another physiologic component to fitness is bone integrity, or how strong and dense our bones are, which is important in preventing osteoporosis (whereby bones become weakened or frail and fractures or breaks are more likely to occur).

A structured exercise program can positively impact physical fitness. The benefits of physical activity and exercise to help you in your goal of having a healthy heart are supported by the research that has shown it prevents occurrences of cardiac events by reducing the incidences of stroke, hypertension, type II diabetes mellitus, colon and breast cancers, osteoporotic fractures, gallbladder disease, obesity, depression and anxiety, and it can prevent an early death.[1]

And it's never too late to start exercising and reap the benefits of increased activity. For example, studies show that individuals who were previously inactive and unfit who become physically active and fit experience lower rates of disease and premature mortality compared to those who continue to remain unfit. This is true for adults of all ages including seniors, confirming there's always time to become physically active to achieve health benefits.[1]

I remember attending a bodybuilding competition and there on the stage was a 76-year-old competitor. He didn't look a day over 50! The only sign that he was in his 70s was the wrinkles on his face that didn't match the average 50-year-old. He was flattered when he was asked for his driver's license as proof of his age. He owed all this to staying at a healthy weight for his height and frame and to exercise, which he swore he began just two years before! He was truly an inspiration to those around him.

Types of Exercise
The three main types of exercise are:
1. Aerobic
2. Anaerobic
3. Flexibility

The main form for cardiovascular endurance is *aerobic exercise*. Examples of aerobic exercise are:
- Walking
- Running
- Bike riding
- Stair climbing
- Rowing
- Cross-country skiing

Aerobic simply means *with oxygen*. As long as oxygen is present, you can continue doing the work, and it remains aerobic. A physical activity that can be performed for a sustained period of time would be aerobic in nature. Jogging and running are examples.

Sprinting and weight training are examples of a second form of exercise – *anaerobic exercise*. This is a form of exercise that does not require oxygen to be present. This is not to say you should hold your breath while sprinting or weight training. There is no exercise performed where it is safe and acceptable to hold your breath. This will dramatically raise your blood pressure to potentially dangerous levels. The point is, theoretically, you could hold your breath and your body would still be able to lift the weight. Conversely, holding your breath while walking on a treadmill won't get you very far for very long.

There are actually two components of anaerobic exercise: muscular strength and muscular endurance. Muscular strength refers to the ability of the muscle to exert force. An example would be lifting a weight for very low repetitions, as in fewer than six times.

Muscular endurance is the muscle's ability to perform many repetitions, such as greater than 12. From a functional standpoint, having increased muscular strength would mean we'd have an easier time lifting heavy grocery bags in the supermarket. Having increased muscular endurance would mean we'd be able to carry those heavy grocery bags across the parking lot to the car with greater ease.

A third type of exercise is *flexibility*. This is defined as the ability to move a joint through its complete range of motion. Maintaining flexibility of all joints helps facilitate joint movement. If a person has poor flexibility and an activity moves the structures of a joint beyond the joint's shortened range of motion, tissue damage can occur.[1]

I'm no stranger to tissue damage as I have torn my hamstrings, triceps and biceps muscles on more than one occasion, related to inflexibility. Unfortunately, there are no set training guidelines for flexibility except to say that stretching may benefit the range of motion of the stretched joint (or joints). However, there is no evidence suggesting that stretching will reduce the incidence of injury or improve performance. In my own practice, I've incorporated stretching which I firmly believe has enabled me to return to exercise with no limitations. Achievements from stretching can diminish within three to four weeks without regular training. A stretching program consisting of 10 to 20 minutes about three times per week appears beneficial for increasing or maintaining range of motion and movement suppleness.[2] (For more information on stretching, see Chapter 8, "Stretching.")

It is not uncommon for new clients of personal trainers/exercise physiologists to be put through a general fitness assessment, prior to beginning a training program. This would give both the professional and the client a baseline to determine how fit the client is and to develop goals to make improvements. In this assessment, all areas of exercise should be addressed: cardiovascular endurance, muscular endurance, muscular strength, and flexibility. In Chapter 7, "Strength Training Exercises," you will be guided to developing a basic workout that will address each of these areas. Chapter 8, as noted above, covers "Stretching." In Chapter 9, "Sample Workouts," you will also see examples of workouts that, under the supervision of your physician, cardiologist, trainer or cardiac rehab nurse, you can adapt to your own situation.

<u>Where Should You Exercise?</u>

The beautiful thing about exercise is that it really can be done anywhere. For aerobic exercise, you simply need to be moving your major muscle groups, such as your legs, for a sustained period of time. As a substitute for walking or running on a treadmill or pedaling on a recumbent bike, you could jump on a trampoline, go for a brisk walk or jog at the beach, or go for a bike ride along a scenic route.

Resistance training and flexibility do not necessarily require a gym membership to perform, either. Free weights and exercise bands can be purchased for your home. Furthermore, I have made it a point to include exercises using common household products as well, reinforcing the fact that it can truly be done anywhere.

<u>Putting Exercise Into Your Weekly Schedule</u>

Over the years, here are the most common barriers to exercise that I have observed, as well as some suggestions for how to overcome each one:

1. Time
2. Cost
3. A disability
4. Lack of motivation
5. Fear

TIME

Making the decision to exercise is a time investment and commitment. Although the act of exercise itself doesn't have to take too long, when you factor in the time it takes in travel to and from the gym, shower, and perhaps socialize a bit, a 30- to 60-minute workout can easily turn into a two-hour burden. For those with a job and family responsibilities, it is not uncommon to put off exercise in order to handle the numerous other daily tasks they may have. Although it is understandable for people to put off exercise to handle these numerous tasks that may take higher priority, this approach is rarely justifiable. In this day and age, there are many solutions to overcome this type of barrier.

For starters, you can develop a time-saving game plan prior to starting the workout. Make a decision on what muscle groups you're going to train. Will you be doing a full-body workout? How about training your upper body on one day and your lower body the next? By knowing what body parts you're going to train and selecting the appropriate exercises prior to beginning the workout, your workout time will be significantly condensed. For new exercisers, hiring a personal trainer to help you design a program or using a program designed in this book can provide the necessary structure to initiate an effective routine.

An exercise log will help keep you on track (see the Appendix for a sample). This is a journal where you not only write down the exercises for the day, but keep track of your sets, repetitions, and weight lifted for each movement. It provides a great way to monitor your progress. You can use your log to determine which part of the day gives you superior workouts. Are you stronger in the morning or evening hours? Are you losing weight as the weeks progress? This is all valuable information that you cannot possibly remember unless you write it down. As you look back at your log from previous workouts, you can ask yourself, "Am I coming closer to accomplishing my goals?" If the answer is no, it's time to make adjustments. Perhaps the solution is doing shorter workouts on a more frequent basis.

Another way to reduce the time invested in the workout is to simply train at home. For under $1,000, you can have a decent exercise bike, a variety of dumbbells and resistance bands, and a stability ball. This will provide a basic setup at home to ensure a thorough and productive workout. A nice advantage is that you wouldn't have to contend with obstacles such as large crowds and traffic.

One other way to reduce the workout time is to go to the gym during off-peak hours. Gyms tend to be busiest between 6:00 and 8:00 am for those exercising before work; 4:00 to 8:00 pm for those exercising after work. Exercising at hours in between these popular times will ensure minimal interruptions and less waiting time to use a particular piece of equipment.

Cost

Cost has been identified as another barrier to exercise. Ten years ago, this excuse may have held more merit; especially with gyms costing anywhere from $40 to $80 per month. But with the advent of more affordable "fitness gyms," rates of $10 to $20 per month have certainly generated a positive response. Even personal training rates at these gyms have become more affordable by the offering of various packages and group plans.

For those who prefer home workouts, purchasing the equipment as mentioned previously for less than $1,000 is another viable option. An added benefit is that this is simply a one-time fee. If this still seems expensive, realize this doesn't need to be purchased all at once. Perhaps start with the purchase of the aerobic equipment, such as a bike or treadmill. Search for bargains, including tag sales, thrift shops, internet websites like eBay, and the "bargain news." You may actually find decent exercise equipment people are trying to get rid of, due to the fact that they never use it anymore. This brings us to our next barrier to exercise ....

DISABILITY

Another barrier to exercise is suffering from a particular disability, leaving handicapped persons feeling as if they are not suited for such physical activity. Examples of these disabilities include being wheelchair bound, suffering from heart disease or respiratory complications, having a fractured extremity, or being severely obese, to name a few. Although exercise in this population can present numerous challenges, the fact is that exercise is not only beneficial for them, but required in many cases to achieve the greatest amount of independence with minimal physical limitations.

Different disabilities require different adjustments in order to exercise safely and successfully. For example, those who are wheelchair bound may have absolutely no use of their lower extremities. As a result, an aerobic exercise for the upper extremities, such as an arm bike, can be used. For resistance training, various machine and free weight exercises are effective. In fact, the professional sport of wheelchair bodybuilding displays some rather impressive, superhero-like physiques.

A fractured extremity may initially require a short layoff from activity, depending on where the fracture is. In many cases, as long as the fracture is stable and secure with a cast, the exerciser can safely and effectively train the opposite limb. In fact, a study in 2004 showed that by continuing to exercise the uninjured limb, the injured limb will experience less muscular atrophy or shrinkage.[3]

Depending on the nature of the heart disease or respiratory complication that exists, exercise can and should be a regular part of daily life. Checking with your doctor is a good idea if you question whether your condition is stable enough to handle such physical stress at this time. These conditions, as well as severe obesity, will be discussed in greater detail later in this book.

LACK OF MOTIVATION

As previously mentioned, the time around the holidays seems to be when people make plans to begin or resume an exercise program. It may be related to the guilt of eating too much of the Thanksgiving and Christmas goodies. It may also have to do with making New Year's resolutions, where losing fat or aiming to lower blood pressure and cholesterol takes precedence. Regardless of the reason, motivation to exercise is high. Unfortunately, something happens shortly after beginning the program, and this motivation deteriorates rather quickly. Although their intentions may be sincere, over half of all who begin an exercise program drop out after six months. So, what is causing this lack of motivation and what can we do to combat this?

One possible explanation is a lack of knowledge regarding how to work out. I see it very often in the gym. I see the stranger roaming around the gym like a little lost soul. He or she may try a particular weight machine, possibly using too much weight and doing jerky-like movements, using too much momentum, which is ineffective in targeting the muscle and potentially dangerous. They would then walk over to another machine, with a stare of bewilderment. They may test the machine out, or wait for another gym member (who may or may not know how to use it correctly) to come over and use it first. After a few weeks of roaming around the gym, feeling as if they don't know what they're doing, they decide to no longer subject themselves to this type of psychological stress.

The key point to realize here is that self-efficacy is the greatest predictor of adherence between three and 12 months after initiation. In other words, if you have confidence in yourself and your ability to perform these exercises in a safe and effective manner, you're more likely to stick with this program for that length of time. For those lacking this confidence, hiring a trainer or using a reference book such as this one can help boost that self-efficacy.

In addition to not knowing what they're doing, this lack of self-efficacy and confidence could be related to the fear of additional health complications due to the stress on their already-injured hearts, among other potential ailments. In my position at a cardiac rehab facility, I've worked one-on-one with many first-time exercisers, in addition to exercise veterans who were simply scared of exercise, fearful of a recurring traumatic episode. Not only is there a physical adjustment for these participants, but a strong psychological adjustment as well. Every success story I can tell (saying "many" would truly be an understatement) comes with one common variable – perseverance. Whether it was a 75-year-old male with awkward gait and little coordination on the treadmill to a 60-year-old female who would never think it possible to press 20-pound dumbbells over her head, perseverance is what led them to success. They never quit on themselves; they set realistic goals and they devoted one hour a day, three days per week until their goals were accomplished. From there, new goals were instinctively set. Throughout the book, you will read about several individuals who persevered and accomplished their personal fitness goals. It was their personal commitment and self-efficacy that truly led them to success.

Fearing that exercise could lead to a second heart attack, stroke, or other health complication is an understandable concern. The fact is exercise is a stress not only to your full body, but specifically to your heart, as well. This particular stress can cause a heart attack. After all, this is one reason why exercise stress tests are performed. It is a way to check for heart problems. Although health complications from exercise can occur, statistics show only one in 2,500 patients will experience a heart attack during a stress test, where the heart rate is potentially pushed to near-maximum levels. It is important to clarify that a typical exercise session wouldn't push your heart to the same extent a stress test would. The positive benefits exercise can bring will reduce your overall risk for heart complications.

A third explanation for the lack of self-efficacy is due to participants' failure to see a positive change from the work they're putting in. For example, if your goal is weight loss and you've recently gained five pounds despite the fact that you've been exercising consistently for the past four weeks, this can be quite discouraging. Or, if your goal is to lower your blood pressure or cholesterol, and a recent physical has shown your blood pressure is higher than ever and your cholesterol is elevated, you may decide exercise is not helping, so why waste the time and money? Again, this is where a personal trainer and/or adopting the principles in this book can lend a helping hand and provide reassurance. Unfortunately, exercise alone may not be enough to give you a "perfect" blood pressure or cholesterol reading. Exercise alone may not be enough to initiate the weight loss. It may take a more aggressive dietary approach combined with exercise to accomplish this goal. The important thing to realize is that confidence is a big factor to compliance. If you lack this confidence, seek help from all available resources (e.g. trainer, nutritionist, instructional book, video, etc.) to overcome the barrier.

One other explanation for poor self-confidence is a lack of social support. Social support is the strongest predictor of long term exercise adherence, described as greater than one year.[4] However, if you are the only one in your social network who is exercising regularly, the people closest to you may not be your biggest supporters. Especially if they are not exercising themselves, they may not be quick to offer encouragement. Furthermore, some of your closest friends may have some pretty unhealthy habits, such as smoking, drinking alcohol in excess, or making frequent unhealthy food choices. If you are in this type of environment, it may be difficult to stay motivated and consistent with your workouts. By contrast, if your friends, romantic partner or relatives are also exercising regularly, especially if you have a training partner to exercise with or friends at the gym, you are more likely to stay motivated and consistent with your workouts.

Even as Mr. CT, I have experienced my fair share of exercise barriers, especially when first starting out. I started exercising at the ripe old age of 13, with a little home-gym setup that I had begged for as a Christmas present. I grew up idolizing such muscular celebrities as Arnold Schwarzenegger, Sylvester Stallone and Hulk Hogan. Weighing 200 pounds at the time motivated me to start exercising, especially since there wasn't much fat-free mass I was carrying. I had a rather large rear-end and belly, which had my back hunched over.

No matter how strong my desire to lose weight and build muscle, I failed to exercise consistently. I hated going downstairs to my cold, dreary basement where the weights were set up. Despite all the equipment that had surrounded me, I failed to see any substantial results. Within three months, the weight set was collecting dust and quickly becoming draped in spider webs.

My desire to exercise was resurrected the following Christmas when I received *The Arnold Schwarzenegger Encyclopedia of Bodybuilding* as a gift. I read the book cover-to-cover and couldn't wait to try out the new exercises I'd learned. Furthermore, I was eager to begin metamorphosing into a replica of the comic-book superhero physiques portrayed in the book. Unfortunately, this new-found enthusiasm again lasted only a few months. My frustration peaked as I quickly fell apart making only minimal improvements. Little did I realize that my biggest problem was following a poor diet.

It wasn't until I was 15 that I had managed to drop over 40 pounds in three months! It didn't happen by training in my basement. It was the rigorous practices of high school football that got my weight under control. With that weight loss, my confidence grew, as well as my desire to achieve the muscular look which brought me right back to my weight set in the basement.

Within several months of training, I found I was utilizing my home equipment less and less. There seemed to be too many distractions around, mainly video games and television. But I overcame these barriers at 16 years of age when I received my driver's license and immediately joined a local gym. I knew that by replacing my comfortable home environment with more of a "working" environment, I would be able to train hard with no interruptions. I quickly became hooked and have been training consistently at a gym ever since.

Over the years of training at various gyms, I've had the pleasure of meeting a variety of knowledgeable weightlifters who gave me the education and motivation I needed to transform myself into a successful bodybuilder. For me, home was not the place where I could routinely push myself. I was able to recognize what my own personal barriers were and made appropriate modifications to foster success. What worked then and still works for me, however, need not be the answer for you. If you are unable or unwilling to go to a gym, whether it is the distance you would need to travel or the cost involved, you can still follow an at-home workout routine and get the benefits of exercise that you are learning about in this book.

FEAR

For others, it is not lack of confidence but actual fear that stops them from exercising. For example, Joyce was 39 when she had her first of two hospitalizations. Although she was previously active, there was no speedy recovery as expected. Ultimately, it was more than her cardiac and skeletal muscles that needed strengthening. Her recovery was due to the strengthening of her spirit. Here is Joyce's story and how she overcame her fear of exercising:

I was four years old when diagnosed with mitral valve prolapse. I had been followed closely by my cardiologist for years to track its progression. By the time I was 39, I was told one side of my heart was enlarged and I would need surgery to repair the valve. This came as a surprise to me because I was really feeling quite well, except for chronic heart palpitations.

Initially after surgery, I was scared of doing damage to the valve. To my knowledge, I had a band around the valve. If I got my heart rate up too high, would the band come apart? This was my greatest fear.

I started cardiac rehab four weeks after my surgery. In addition to being afraid to elevate my heart rate, I also feared I wouldn't be able to do my normal physical activities again. I was getting so tired and short of breath with what little exercise I did, I couldn't last more than 50 seconds of aerobic activity without needing a break.

I used to have a regular exercise program, pedaling like a champ on the elliptical walker at my local gym. It took several weeks, but I gradually progressed to five full minutes without stopping. With the rehab staff being so friendly and patient with me, I felt a good sense of security and trusted they would keep me safe. Not only did I stay safe, but I managed to get myself to my previous 30 minutes of continuous pedaling on that dreaded elliptical. My confidence was soaring by the time I had graduated.

For the next five years, I did well with exercise and following a heart-healthy diet, which I had also learned in rehab. I must confess my diet was not really structured before I had started. Through the educational classes, I learned how to read labels and eat a low fat, low sodium, and low cholesterol diet. My kids, who were 16, six, and five at the time, were such a great support, were willing to try their mom's healthy foods, such as asparagus! Although my husband loves his fried foods, he was a strong supporter as well.

It wasn't until one day at 44 years of age that my fears resurfaced. I remember like it was yesterday. I had just finished having dinner with friends at the casino when I became short of breath while climbing stairs. I got so scared and suddenly passed out.

When I had regained consciousness, I was in the process of being transported to the hospital by helicopter. At the hospital, it was discovered I had a pulmonary embolism, which I later learned was a blood clot in my lung.

Once the clot was dissolved and I was discharged from the hospital, I had the opportunity to do another round of cardiac rehab sessions. This time, I was even more afraid to exercise. Part of this fear was due to having a stress test a couple of weeks before my traumatizing experience. Although I passed with flying colors, I was thinking that stressing my heart at that time led to my blood clot. If I were to "push myself" again, would I develop another blood clot?

Similar to the last go-around, I had begun cardiac rehab four weeks after discharge. Although the nurses were very encouraging, I was still fearful of developing another clot. What added to the intense anxiety was listening to the sound of flying helicopters very frequently, being that I conveniently lived very close to a major helicopter manufacturing plant.

Not only did the rehab staff help me regain my confidence with exercise, they had referred me to a therapist to help me deal with post-traumatic stress disorder. Honestly, it took a good three years before I really felt confident in my ability to push myself.

Like the saying goes, "Time heals all wounds." I realize that I am protected with daily blood thinners that I faithfully take. I am proud to say I am remaining consistent with all of my workouts and feel better *than ever! I can now sleep peacefully at night without reliving the episode every time I hear a chopper pass by.*

One thing I have learned through this whole ordeal is that I needed to push through my fear of exercise. I had to have confidence and belief in myself that I could get over this and feel better. I am proud to say I am finally there!

Taking all of this in, reflect on your own personal barriers. Identify them and come up with a plan to combat them. If you lack the social support, find a training partner you can exercise with. This companion should have similar goals and be willing to exercise at a mutually convenient time. If you lack the confidence and self-efficacy, choose a training partner who is knowledgeable and consistent with exercise, refer to the workouts in this book, or hire a trainer. If you feel time is an issue, plan shorter, more frequent workouts. Find the schedule that works best for you, whether it's as early as 5:00 am or as late as 9:00 pm. With certain disabilities, working closely with a registered clinical exercise physiologist (RCEP) can provide the necessary guidelines and education needed to implement a safe and effective program. Whatever barriers exist, if you are willing to overcome them, the necessary resources are available to you. Use this in good health; for good health.

Joining a Gym or Cardiac Health Program

No time is more popular to begin an exercise program than right after the New Year. As early as January 2, the local gyms are packed with newly motivated exercisers, psyched and ready to make up for lost time. Some are brand new to exercise, requiring a thorough orientation by a fairly fit and friendly trainer. For many others, exercise is nothing new. They don't feel as if they ever left the gym, despite the six- or seven-month layoff they may have experienced.

Whatever time of year you are picking up this book, there is no time like the present to start your new commitment to exercising. Avoid the "trap" of feeling that you should wait until the New Year to make a fresh start. After checking with your physician and getting clearance to exercise, why not start right away?

Exercising at Home

As stated earlier, exercise does not have to be done at a gym in order for it to be effective. Every so often, I have clients in cardiac rehab who complain about how boring exercise is, just walking on the *conveyor belt* we call a treadmill. My challenge is to find what physical activities they do enjoy and what they are willing to do as a realistic alternative to "traditional" exercise.

I've worked with tennis players, badminton players, golfers (not riding in carts) and swimmers, to name a few. Although these sports enthusiasts may not keep their heart rates elevated for 30 to 60 minutes continuously, they will have frequent periods where their heart rates are elevated, much as if they were engaged in *interval training* (See Chapter 6).

Gardening can be a fun and beneficial form of physical activity. This involves squatting and pulling on a regular basis.

A coworker of mine really enjoys dancing. Her physician never fails to remind her that she needs to lose about 30 pounds for her overall health. I'm pleased to say she is finally going to the gym on a regular basis. What's suddenly keeping her compliant isn't the lovely selection of bikes, treadmills and weight machines. It is the Zumba™ dance classes that she's participating in that have led to her 17-pound weight loss in three months!

It's not that she is avoiding the traditional gym machines. She's merely mixing up her workouts, where she includes dancing several times a week, which she really enjoys. She knows that it's only a matter of time before she loses the additional 13 pounds.

Exercise should be enjoyable if you expect to be compliant with it. Use your regular household chores, sporting activities, and other recreational pursuits to get your heart rate up and burn some calories. Think of what items you have at home that could be an alternative to dumbbells if inaccessible. (You will find some examples of exercises in Chapter 7, "Strength Training Exercises," using household items to get you started). Be creative, and most importantly, have fun!

Chapter 6

Aerobics: Frequency, Duration and Intensity

We've already discussed the importance of regular aerobic (cardiovascular) exercise to maintain a healthy heart and strengthen a deconditioned or weakened heart. Many people include aerobic training in their regimen, but often without a strategy. They may be doing cardiovascular exercise with the purpose of losing weight, but fail to eat right and end up quitting their exercise routine, due to lack of progress. Or perhaps cardiovascular exercise is done for a strong and healthy heart. But if done too infrequently, the heart-strengthening benefits of aerobics will not be achieved. The goal of this chapter is to help you design an effective cardiovascular program to achieve your exercise objectives. We will look at the three factors that you need to consider for your optimal exercise program: frequency, duration and intensity (FDI).

Frequency

> *Rule of thumb: An effective cardiovascular conditioning regimen should be performed at least three times a week, on nonconsecutive days. Further benefits can be achieved by more than three sessions per week, but three is the bare minimum.*

Those with special needs, such as those who are trying to lose weight, may benefit from more than one session per day. However, rather than doing two or more exercise sessions in one day, and not making the time to exercise the rest of the week, it is better to go for once a day, at least three times a week, as a minimum. This is based on studies that show the deconditioning process whereby your fitness level begins to decline after about three days of inactivity.[1] That is the rationale for doing your exercise routine on nonconsecutive days. The bottom line: The longer you go without doing aerobics, the greater the deconditioning you can expect. Unfortunately, deconditioning often results in a lack of motivation for continuing your exercise program in the long run, since your body goes back to the way it was before you started exercising and gaining stamina and muscle strength. Inconsistency in your exercise program, and the resultant deconditioning, can lead you to give up completely. So spacing out your exercise sessions, so your frequency is lower but your consistency is greater, will usually give you the better short- and long-term results.

One of the things that come to mind when I think of the word *frequency* is the poor attendance I see in cardiac rehab, especially in the summer vacationing months. I understand that work and home-responsibilities can interfere with exercise sessions on certain days and times. However, my clients are free to exercise on their own at home or at a local gym. I just advise them to work no harder on their own than they would in cardiac rehab, where they are closely monitored. With most hotels and cruise ships offering on-site fitness centers, there are no excuses for not dedicating some time for exercise while traveling. I can usually spot those individuals who exercised less than three times per week. They fail to make noticeable progress, and every workout seems to be just as challenging as the previous one. Their speed and incline settings on the treadmill never change, nor does their wattage on the bike improve. I preach to them how three days per week is the bare minimum to exercise and greater gains can be experienced with additional sessions per week. Those following the guidelines of at least three days per week surely feel the difference when they have missed a session or two.

I remember one participant in cardiac rehab who went on a two-week cruise. Prior to his trip, he was fairly compliant, hardly ever missing a workout. After his cruise, I had not seen him for another month. When asked about his six-week absence, his reply was, "There is no excuse. I just got busy with other things." Unfortunately, his busy work did not include exercise, nor did he visit the fitness center on the cruise ship.

There was no need to lecture him about the importance of frequency in his workouts. The fact that he was huffing and puffing at a lower-than-usual setting on the treadmill was evidence enough for him. It took about three weeks of regular attendance three days per week and additional sessions at his local gym for him to return to his conditioning level before his vacation. He learned his lesson, albeit the hard way.

Duration

Now that we've covered the frequency of aerobics, I will address another key concern, namely, duration. The American College of Sports Medicine recommends 30-60 minutes of physical activity on most, if not all, days of the week. For cardiovascular benefits, you should aim for at least 30 minutes.[2] No greater benefits will be achieved beyond 60 minutes of *continuous* aerobic activity, but the risk of injury increases.[3]

> *Rule of thumb: Aim for a minimum of 30 minutes for each workout and a maximum of 60 minutes. Less than 30 minutes per day will not give you the best cardiovascular benefits. More than 60 minutes will not provide any greater gains but there is an enhanced risk of injury.*

Intensity

Intensity is the third important issue. How hard should you be working out when you are doing aerobics? One way to determine this is by taking a percentage of your maximum heart rate. For a general cardiovascular conditioning program, the ACSM recommends a target heart rate between 60% and 85% of your age-predicted maximum. An age-predicted estimated maximum heart rate has generally been calculated as 220 minus your age. So for a 50-year-old, the age-predicted maximum heart rate would be 170 bpm. Taking 60-85% of 170 will give us a target heart rate range of 102-144.5 (145) bpm.

A recent study has shown a more accurate estimation of an age-predicted maximum heart rate.[4] In this study, researchers found greater accuracy in the equation: 207 minus 0.7 times your age.

Using this formula in the same 50-year-old individual, our new age-predicted maximum heart rate would be 172 bpm. As a result, our new target heart rate range would be 103-146 bpm. As you can see, both formulas give roughly the same range. Therefore, use whichever formula is easiest to remember.

These equations work well for the healthy population, but do not work so well for those taking medications that slow the heart rate, such as beta blockers. For this population, a better measurement of intensity is the rate of perceived exertion (RPE) scale:

0) Nothing at all   (basically asleep)
1) Very weak   (light warm-up)
2) Weak   (warm-up)
3) Moderate   (muscles are worked, but can increase intensity)
4) Somewhat strong   (muscles are worked; handling intensity)
5) Strong   (breathing faster but handling intensity)
6)
7) Very strong   (can't carry conversation; can't continue long)
8)
9) Extremely strong   (need to stop; can't catch your breath)
10) Maximum   (most intense pain ever; must stop now)

This scale is frequently used during stress tests, as well as in cardiac rehabilitation centers. It gives health professionals a clear understanding of how hard the patient feels he or she is working. A good target number is to aim between 3 and 5 on the RPE scale. Remember: Aerobic exercise means *with oxygen*. As long as oxygen is present, you can continue to do the work, such as walking on the treadmill. Staying at a range of 3 to 5 on the RPE scale should be sufficient to keep oxygen present.

Whether or not you are on heart medications that slow your heart rate, the RPE scale is probably the best guide of intensity to use. You may have those occasional days where even 60% of your age-predicted maximum heart rate is too much. Instead of reaching exhaustion or risking injury, just take that particular session as a lower-intensity session, using the RPE scale as your guide. You might be surprised how high your heart rate can climb after 20 minutes or so at a lower intensity. You may find you've reached 65% of your estimated maximum heart rate, but it took 20 minutes or so to get there. The important thing is to do what you can do on that given day. Doing *something* is usually better than doing nothing.

An exercise science term worth mentioning is *MET* level. MET is short for *metabolic equivalents*. It represents milliliters of oxygen per kilogram of bodyweight per minute. It's a measurement of the amount of oxygen your body is able to utilize at a given time. It's basically a fitness measurement, wherein the higher the intensity of exercise, the higher the MET level, thus, the higher the fitness level. For example, an average 200-pound individual working out on a stair climber at level 1 may be working at 4 METs. If another 200-pound individual is exercising at level 5 on the stair climber, he or she would be working at about 8 METs. It should be obvious which individual is in better cardiovascular shape.

Because MET levels can be increased through regular training, there is hope for all individuals to get in better shape. In fact, studies show that those in the worst shape tend to make the greatest improvements! So don't be discouraged if you are "out of shape" or you haven't exercised in a very long time. You want to, of course, see your doctor or cardiologist and get the okay to start exercising regularly. Once you do, you may be astounded at the progress you make!

You can keep track of your progress by simply keeping an exercise log, writing down what speed and incline you've achieved on the treadmill, or what level you've accomplished on the bike, Stairmaster, etc. (A sample blank log is provided in the Appendix). In fact, many aerobic machines have a button you can press to calculate what MET level you're currently exercising at. Ways to achieve improvements are by increasing the duration of exercise (i.e. 30 minutes to 40 minutes, etc.), frequency (i.e. three days per week to five days per week, etc.), or intensity (i.e. MET level). Similar to strength training, where getting used to lifting a heavier weight will get you stronger, walking at a faster speed or steeper incline will improve your fitness level. This can only further strengthen your heart.

No matter what the activity, every exerciser sooner or later becomes familiar with the phrase "hitting a plateau." A plateau in the exercise world is when you reach a point in your exercise program where you are no longer seeing improvement in one or more aspects of your physical fitness (strength, endurance, flexibility). This can be explained by Hans Selye's GAS (general adaptation syndrome) principle, which the Canadian biologist and endocrinologist used to describe how the human body reacts to stress. He identified three stages of an individual's responds to stress (Fig. 17). Years later, Selye's GAS principle was applied to exercise training by Dr. John Garhammer, professor of biomechanics at California State University.[5]

In the *alarm phase*, the body experiences a new physical stress. The initial response is soreness, stiffness and a small decline in performance. This could last a few days to a few weeks, depending on the intensity of the stress and conditioning of the exerciser.

In the *resistance phase*, the body now becomes adapted to the physical stress applied. This is where you will see a steady improvement in performance until you reach a plateau. If the stress persists for an extended period, the exerciser will likely reach the *exhaustion phase*. Here, many of the symptoms from the *alarm phase* return. The difference is that the exerciser won't rebound as quickly. He or she may experience fatigue, weakness, excessive soreness, a decreased immune system resulting in a higher susceptibility to illness, and potential injury. Every effort should be made to avoid this stage. This is where breaking the monotony in your workouts, not training too hard for too long, and adequate nutrition, rest, and sleep are crucial. To make further progress, be creative in finding new ways to stress the body, such as going for a bike ride outside several days per week instead of a brisk walk on the treadmill every day. Change the order of exercises in your weight training regimen, and vary the number of sets and repetitions.

In my personal routine, for example, I have a "heavy week," where I perform six sets consisting of 12, 10, 8, 8, 6, and 6 repetitions. I gradually increase the weight until I select the heaviest weight I can lift for two sets of six repetitions. My next week is a "light week," where I perform four sets of 10 repetitions. Every four to six weeks, I will substitute a "super-light" week, where I perform four sets of 25, 20, 15, and 10 repetitions. Because of the diversity of my training on a weekly basis, neither my body nor my mind gets bored or tired, keeping my workouts fresh and stimulating.

Figure 17: Hans Selye's General Adaptation Syndrome

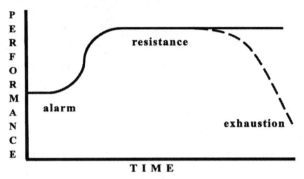

One such method to increase your MET level from a cardiovascular perspective is interval training.[5]

This is done by exercising at a low intensity (no greater than 3 on RPE scale) for one minute, then increasing the intensity to a high intensity level (6 or 7 on RPE scale) for 1 minute, then back to low intensity for one minute, then high intensity for another minute, etc. This would go on for no longer than 20 minutes. No greater benefits are achieved after such time. If you are just starting out, you can make it less challenging by doing two minutes at a low intensity with one minute at a higher intensity; even five minutes at a lower intensity with 30 seconds to one minute of a higher intensity.

Interval training should be done no more than three days per week for less than or equal to 20 minutes per session. You can compare interval training to weight training in that in order to increase strength, you need to be able to lift a heavier weight. Let's say you can bench press 225 pounds for eight repetitions, with seemingly no improvements in several weeks. To shock the body, you'll put 275 pounds on the bench and may get only three repetitions. By attempting the weight several times for the next few weeks, three repetitions turn into four, which turn into six, which eventually may lead to 10 repetitions!

Interval training works in a similar way, whereby level 6 on the stair climber for one minute will turn into 90 seconds at level 6, which will lead to three minutes at level 6 and, ultimately, 30 minutes at level 6!

If you choose interval training as your method of exercise, stay safe by training within your target heart-rate range. If you're on heart-rate-lowering medications, get to know what range you are comfortably in with an RPE of 3-5. Stay within that heart-rate range, and you should be just fine.

Another important point to discuss is what setting to enter in on the cardiovascular machines. Many aerobic machines have different programs you can enter in on the console. You can enter in a fat-burning program or interval option, similar to what I had just mentioned. I caution you with these settings, as the machine will adjust the level of intensity on its own. I must admit I am not a fan of this because the machine is unaware of how you're feeling that day, or whether or not you're taking medications that lower your heart rate. The machine may bump up the MET level to a point you cannot handle. To avoid this, use "manual" as the option of choice. This will enable you to control the machine and adjust the level of intensity as you see fit.

Exercising to prevent a heart attack or as a strategy to regain your health after one occurs

As you know by now, I am a strong advocate for including exercise in your week's activities as a way to lower your risk of a heart attack as well as a way to deal with stress and to help you with your weight goals. For some, however, exercise is introduced into their routine only after a heart attack or "event" occurs. This is what happened with 46-year-old Jane*, who reluctantly began an exercise program after she had a heart event. I worked with Jane for three-and-a-half months in the rehab center and later she agreed to let me interview her about her experiences. I think you may find her story touches on many of the resistances you may be having to exercise, such as a fear of exercising. How she overcame that fear, and the benefits of exercise in her life, will, I hope, be inspiring to you:

I was 46 years old when I had my [heart] event. While walking my eight-year-old autistic daughter to her bus stop one morning, I had noticed my chest was pounding and I was becoming short of breath. The bus stop is at the top of a fairly steep hill, one that never bothered me previously. Although I don't exercise and am considered moderately obese, I found it a bit concerning that I was becoming so winded from a short walk uphill.

After a couple of days battling these symptoms, I decided to go to an urgent care center. After interpreting my EKG, the doctor advised me to go to the hospital because it appeared questionable.

At the hospital, the cardiologist scheduled me for a stress test two days later. It was then that I was informed I had an 80% blockage in my left anterior descending artery. He told me I would need to have an angioplasty and stent placed to open up the blockage. He scheduled the procedure for three days later and told me to basically be on bed rest until then.

It was the longest three days of my life. Part of me just wanted it done immediately. The other part of me was scared to death, worrying about what would happen to me, as well as my family.

After the procedure, everything seemed to hit me at once. I now had all of these new medications to take. I was previously taking only a women's multi-vitamin. My diet had to change drastically. Everything that was "white" had to be replaced with "brown." I loved eating white bread and white rice. Now, everything had to be whole grain -- whole wheat bread and brown rice – disgusting! What was especially hard was Thanksgiving that year. You see, I was discharged from the hospital the day before Thanksgiving. Having not realized how serious my situation was, my mother insisted on me coming to her place as was the tradition. Not only did I need the energy to make the trip from Connecticut to New York, but I also had to make my favorite dish – macaroni and cheese!

All was well for that day, but it was especially hard for me to just eat plain white turkey meat and vegetables.

In addition to medication and dietary changes, my cardiologist referred me to cardiac rehabilitation, which I began three weeks later.

I was initially very nervous about the program. I was worried about what the nurses and exercise physiologist would make me do and whether or not my heart would be able to handle it. I remember during my first session, I was listening to the education topic of the day. I was sitting with much older participants surrounding a large table. I could sense all of these eyes staring right at me, wondering, "What is she doing here? She's too young to be here!"

Not only was I scared, but felt ashamed.

The first couple of weeks were the hardest for me, as I was trying to become acclimated to the exercise routine. I was afraid I would over-stress my heart. It wasn't until the third week that I started to get into a comfort zone. I felt more confident in my ability to "push myself" without fearing I'd be back in the hospital. I trusted the staff would keep me safe and know how to help me progress safely.

Before long, I was feeling really good after a typical exercise session. No longer was I laboring while walking my daughter up the hill to her bus stop. I even managed to take off 20 pounds through exercise and making the necessary dietary changes.

By the time I had graduated the cardiac rehab program, I had joined a local fitness center and Weight Watchers™ nutrition program.

Overall, my family has been very supportive. I have a loving husband who is big into eating healthy and regular exercise. Every so often, he would get on my case if I skipped an exercise session or two. My 17-year-old son has been a real trooper. He was 15 at the time and was initially concerned I was overdoing it with my daily household chores. As he saw my confidence increase, his confidence in me similarly increased.

My daughter has been an angel throughout the whole experience, although she can be a handful, as any parent of a child with autism can relate to. My mother initially did not realize how life-threatening my blockage was. As time went on, she understood and was very supportive. Being that she used to be a chef, she doesn't hesitate to send over her specialty cakes and cookies. Neither myself nor my kids need such gestures because her love and affection are always felt.

But keeping up with your exercise routine, as well as eating well, can sometimes fall by the wayside. Perhaps you can relate to what Jane shares about herself and how it became necessary to restart her exercise and healthy diet programs:

Now that it has been two years since my event, I shamefully admit I have fallen off of the wagon. Although I continue to pay my monthly fee to the fitness center, I have not been going. Both stress and time-management have been my greatest barriers. In addition to being exhausted from cooking, cleaning the house, and parenting responsibilities, I also work from home. I am a writer who spends no less than five hours a day sitting at a computer. I can spend several more hours sitting at a table sewing various fabrics, since I am a fashion designer. With all of these time-consuming but necessary sedentary activities, I've regrettably neglected an additional important responsibility – exercise. To make matters worse, I am an emotional eater. Once I get stressed, I don't hesitate to reach for the food cabinet.

One of the great things about being asked to share my story is [that] it forced me to reflect on my own exercise habits of late and rejuvenated me to get back in shape. Another positive influence for me was watching my neighbor's dog for a week. For those seven days, I had an exercise partner who demanded we go for our "power walks" two times a day. It's funny how we don't think twice about taking our dogs out for their daily walks but neglect our own.

I'm proud to say I'm now back on track with my diet and exercise program. To avoid binge-ing when stressed out, I now reach for a large bowl of low-calorie salad. This allows me to munch guilt-free. To stay consistent with exercise, I go to the gym bright and early in the morning. This enables me to finish before I get bombarded with work and household chores.

My advice for the young ladies out there is to take care of your body while you are young. When you are in your teens and 20s, you feel you can get away with eating and drinking what you want and not exercising. As you age, your body changes. It hit me like a ton of bricks when I had my heart event. Be sure to keep moving!

Warm up and cool down

I cannot bring this chapter to a close without mentioning the importance of a warm-up and cool-down. It's never really a good idea to take a resting heart and suddenly demand an immediate high level of work for the next 30-or-so minutes. This is an unnecessary stress to the heart muscle. It is similar to lying on a bench and doing a maximum-weight bench press without a warm-up set. It is an injury waiting to happen. Be kind to your heart and respect the need to slowly increase your heart rate over a three- to five-minute period.

The cool-down period is no less important. Three to five minutes of a lower intensity should be performed at the end of the session as well. A good rule to follow is to warm up and cool down at less than or equal to 50% of the intensity you are working at.

In review:

- Perform at least three days per week of aerobics on nonconsecutive days.

This will prevent an unproductive four-day rest period. Keep in mind that aerobics can safely be performed as often as seven days per week.

- Be sure to warm up before every session, followed by a cool-down at the end.

For maximum cardiovascular benefits, exercise at a moderate intensity (60-85% of maximum heart rate or 3-5 on RPE scale) for 30-60 minutes per session.[6] If you need to divide your sessions up into two or three sessions of 10 or 15 minutes, similar cardiovascular benefits will be achieved.[7,8] In Chapter 10, I will discuss examples of training routines that focus on specific populations such as people with diabetes, arthritis and so forth.

To break a plateau, you can experiment with interval training, being sure to keep your heart rate in a safe range.

In the next two chapters, Chapter 7, "Strength Training Exercises," and Chapter 8, "Stretching," I'll explore this key information; you will find the exercises that are described illustrated with one or two photographs so you can more easily visualize what each exercise should look like when you are performing it.

Chapter 7

Strength Training Exercises: Exploring our Muscle Groups

In this chapter, I will describe, and then show, through one or two paragraphs, key exercises that you can do to improve your stamina, burn calories and enhance your flexibility. In this chapter you will learn about, and see illustrations for, exercises for your:

- Chest
- Back
- Legs
- Abdominal muscles
- Shoulders
- Arms (triceps, biceps, and forearms)

Workout clothing should be loose fitting. It puzzles me when I see exercisers wearing tight jeans to work out in. I don't see how it can be comfortable, nor can I imagine squatting in them. For me, that is a tear waiting to happen (clothing tear, not muscle). I would recommend shorts, sweatpants or nylon warm-up pants. A comfortable T-shirt, tank top or sweatshirt would be fine. If you are generally cold, you may want to consider wearing layers, such as a T-shirt under a sweatshirt. You will most likely get hot as your body temperature rises with exercise.

Comfortable sneakers should be worn for walking, jogging or running. Be sure to get sneakers properly fitted from a salesman at a retail shoe store. I remember having painful blisters at the bottom of my feet while playing tennis in college. The mistake I had made was trying to wear sneakers that were fashionable. Unfortunately, what was fashionable was not comfortably fitting. After wearing three pairs of socks to cushion my blistery feet, I decided to surrender and have a professional shoe salesman point me in the right direction with footwear.

As I mentioned in previous chapters, if you have an opportunity to work with an exercise physiologist or *qualified* personal trainer with a nationally recognized certification, I encourage you to take it. They will reinforce proper form for all exercises with you. If not, however, you can use my detailed instructions to take you step-by-step through every exercise. Exercises can be performed in a gym, or at home using free weights or common everyday household items. You will see examples of this in various photos using paint cans, chairs and laundry detergent bottles.

If you have any sort of musculoskeletal abnormality or injury, be sure to stay away from any movement that causes you pain (refer to Chapter 11 to learn more about this). Whether you decide to work with a trainer or do these exercises on your own, be sure to obtain clearance from your physician that it is indeed safe for you to partake in an exercise program.

Regarding rest periods, I would suggest two to three minutes rest per set of each exercise. Of course, when working larger muscles such as your legs, you may need slightly longer rest periods in order to catch your breath. No matter what training level you are at (beginner, intermediate or advanced), your breathing rate should return to just about normal before attempting another set. As you move up to the advanced level, you may want to shorten your rest periods to as little as 60 seconds between sets. This can really elevate the intensity, especially if you wear a stopwatch to keep accurate time.

Regarding the duration of your workouts, the sample exercise routines I have provided for you would take approximately 45 to 60 minutes to complete. If you plan on doing aerobic exercise during the same workout, I strongly recommend doing your weight training while you are fresh and strong. It is fine to do a five- to 10-minute warm-up on a bike or treadmill to get your heart rate and body temperature up, but don't plan on staying on there for the long haul. You will perform better for your weight training and aerobics if you start with the lifting and finish with the aerobics. Of course, you can surely pick a different time of the day to do either aerobics or resistance training. That's the beauty of exercise: the choice is entirely yours.

A note about weight training:
When first starting out a weight training program, I recommend using lighter weights for higher repetitions. This will give you practice and familiarity performing the exercise, as well as strengthening the tendons, which connect your muscles to bones. The muscles can get strong fast, but you are only as strong as your weakest link. To develop tendon strength as well as muscle strength, I usually spend the first four weeks of starting or resuming a weight training regimen with 10 to 15 repetitions per set. Depending on how you feel, you can perform anywhere from one to four working sets when first starting out. A working set is one in which you pick a weight heavy enough where you can just barely make the number of repetitions you are striving for, with perfect form. It is not where you are blue in the face, grunting out loud and straining hard. There is no purpose for that in any weight training program. As you move

on to the intermediate and advanced routines, you will notice the repetitions drop to as little as six. It is expected that you will now select a weight you can lift for six repetitions. The intensity will, therefore, increase.

It is always a good idea to do one to two warm-up sets, where you select a weight that is light and non-challenging to simply "wake up" the muscles before moving on to the heavier weights. Perform a good 12 to 15 non-challenging repetitions here.

CHEST

The chest (also known as the pectoral muscles) serves two basic functions. It enables us to press out and pull inward. It makes up some of the larger muscles of our body. As a result, we tend to be stronger with chest exercises. Below are exercises that target the chest.

Warning: I must warn those who have had open heart surgery within the past 12 weeks of starting an exercise program that it would be best to avoid these exercises to allow the midsternal incision ample time to heal. After 12 weeks, it should be safe to introduce these exercises, but be sure to consult with your cardiologist and/or internist and get his or her permission to begin one or more of these exercises.

Chest Exercises

<u>Push up against counter</u>

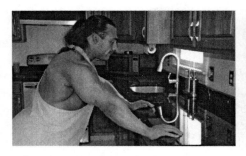 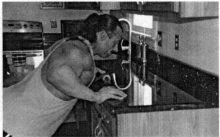

This exercise will benefit your chest, triceps and the front of your shoulders.

- Stand with feet close together, keeping abs tight and hands shoulder-width apart, against the edge of the counter.
- Begin by slowly lowering your chest toward the counter edge.

- From there, press up forcefully, allowing your arms to almost completely straighten.
- Keep repetitions continuous, with no rest between the lowering and rising phases.

Number of repetitions:

Beginner: 10 to 12

Intermediate: 12 to 15

Advanced: failure (perform as many repetitions as possible, until you can no longer complete the movement with perfect form)

Cable chest press

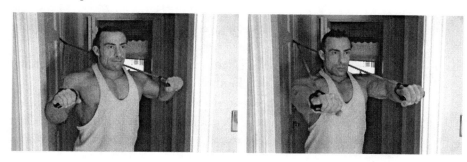

This exercise will benefit your chest, triceps and the front of your shoulders.

- Attach an exercise band or tubing to a pole or door.
- Grasp tubing in each hand and stand far enough away from attachment site to allow tension on the chest muscle.
- Begin by having your arms in a bent position and forcefully press arms outward, straightening them.
- Focus on squeezing the chest muscles as you press out.
- Slowly lower your arms to the starting bent position.
- Keep repetitions continuous, with no rest during the pressing or lowering phases.

Number of repetitions:

Beginner: 10 to 12

Intermediate: 12 to 15

Advanced: failure

Cable chest fly

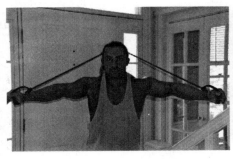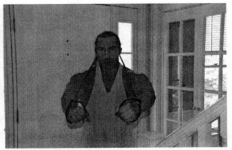

This exercise will benefit your chest, with modest recruitment of your biceps.

- Attach an exercise band or tubing to a pole or door at an area above your head.
- Grasp tubing in each hand and stand far enough from the door, facing away, to allow tension on the chest muscles.
- Have your hands extended out away from your body.
- Begin by having a slight bend in your elbows and squeeze your chest muscles as you bring your hands as close together as possible without touching.
- Pretend you are giving somebody a big bear hug.
- Slowly return your arms to a starting position and repeat for the required repetitions. Squeeze your chest muscles as you perform the movement.

Number of repetitions:
Beginner: 10 to 12
Intermediate: 12 to 15
Advanced: failure

Dumbbell chest press on Swiss ball

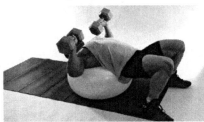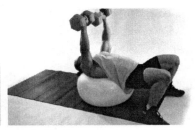

This exercise will benefit your chest, triceps, and the front of your shoulders, along with your core stabilizer muscles (abdominals, obliques and lower back).

- Sit on a Swiss ball (which you can purchase from most sports stores as well as fitness sections of department stores) with a dumbbell in each hand.
- Walk your feet forward as you slide back on the ball to a starting position with your upper back and neck supported against the ball. This should be a relatively comfortable position.
- Begin the movement by slowly pressing the dumbbells up to an end position of having your arms straight with a slight bend in the elbows, ensuring constant tension on the chest muscles.
- Slowly return the dumbbells to the starting position, obtaining a comfortable stretch.

Number of repetitions:
Beginner: 10 to 12
Intermediate: 8 to 10
Advanced: 6 to 10

<u>Dumbbell chest fly on Swiss ball</u>

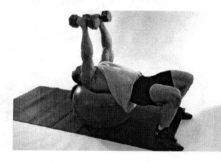 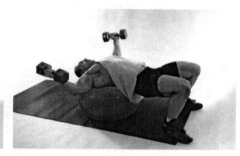

This exercise will benefit your chest, with modest recruitment of your biceps, in addition to your core stabilizer muscles.

- Sit on a Swiss ball with dumbbells in each hand.
- Walk your feet forward as you slide your back on to the ball to a starting position with your upper back and neck fully supported against the ball. This should be a relatively comfortable position. The starting position is having the dumbbells pressed out with palms facing each other, with a slight bend in the elbows.
- Lower your arms until parallel to the floor, obtaining a gentle stretch in the chest muscles.

- Focus on squeezing your chest muscles as you raise your arms back to the starting position. (Envision yourself giving somebody a big bear hug.)

Number of repetitions:

Beginner: 10 to 12

Intermediate: 12 to 15

Advanced: 8 to 12

Kneeling cable pullover

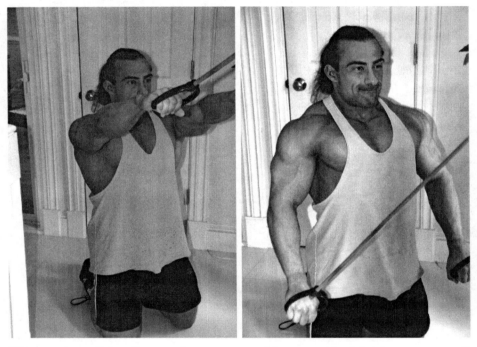

This exercise will benefit your chest, triceps and latissimus dorsi (wide component of your upper and middle back).

- Attach an exercise band or tubing to the top of the door with door attachment (small loop that attaches in a closed door). Be sure to use a door strong enough to handle such resistance.
- Kneel down on the floor facing away from the door and move forward, increasing the distance between yourself and the door.

- Lean forward slightly and grasp the handles with arms up straight. Palms should face outward.
- Begin movement by bringing handles down to shoulder length, being sure to keep arms straight.
- Focus on squeezing your back muscles as you bring the handles down.
- Slowly return the handles to a starting position and complete all required repetitions.

Number of repetitions:

Beginner: 10 to 12

Intermediate: 12 to 15

Advanced: failure (perform as many repetitions as possible, until you can no longer complete the movement with perfect form)

<u>Pushup</u>

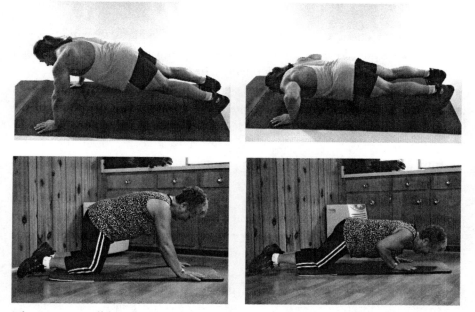

This exercise will benefit your chest, triceps and the front of your shoulders.

- Begin by getting down on all four limbs, keeping your arms and legs straight. The balls of your feet should be in contact with the ground. If you lack the strength to handle pushups in this position, you could perform them with your knees in contact with the ground. As you get stronger, you can progress to the traditional form of pushup with the balls of your feet planted on the ground.

- The distance between your hands should be about shoulder-width apart.
- Start the motion by lowering your chest toward the ground, bending your elbows.
- Just before touching the floor with your chest, press up, straightening out your arms as you come up. The lowering phase should be done slower than the rising phase.

Number of repetitions:

Beginner: 10 to 12

Intermediate: 12 to 15 repetitions to failure

Advanced: failure (perform as many repetitions as possible, until you can no longer complete the movement with perfect form)

BACK

Similar to your chest, your back serves two basic functions in your body: it enables you to pull down and pull in. An example of pulling down is doing a pull-up. An example of pulling in is rowing a boat.

The back comprises a large muscle group, making up the latissimus dorsi (a.k.a. "lats"), rhomboids, trapezius, and spinal erectors. You can think of the lats and rhomboids making up the width and thickness of the upper and middle back. The trapezius muscle connects the upper back to the neck. The spinal erectors are muscles of the lower back, which function in keeping the body balanced by keeping the spine erect.

In 2007, about 12% of U.S. adults ages 18 and older reported having back problems. About 19 million adults reported receiving treatment for back pain that same year. A total of $4.5 billion was spent on prescription medications to treat back problems in adults. This is clearly a problem that needs correction.[1]

Whether to treat back pain or prevent it from happening in the first place, the following exercises can be used to strengthen not only your back, but also the smaller stabilizer muscles that can help take stress off an injured area. The following exercises will enforce proper body mechanics, helping you lift heavy objects with perfect form. The same form you will learn in picking up a heavy weight can be applied to picking up an object from the floor, even if it is as light as a piece of paper. Using proper body mechanics (flawless form) is crucial to preventing back injury.

Back Exercises

<u>Standing cable row</u>

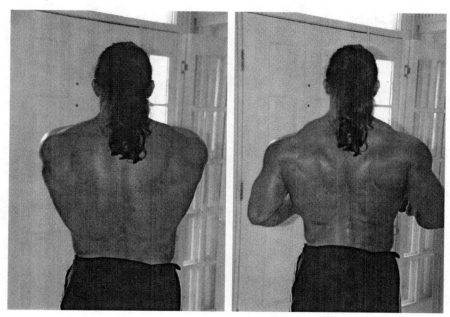

This exercise will benefit the upper and middle portions of your back, along with your biceps.

- Stand with an exercise band or tubing tied to a secure bar at your midline, so that two sides of the band are grasped in your hands.
- Stand back far enough to ensure arms and back muscles are well stretched.
- Begin the movement by driving the elbows back as far as possible, maximally contracting the back muscles.
- Keep your back straight as you return to the starting position, achieving a good stretch in the back and arms.

Number of repetitions:
Beginner: 10 to 12
Intermediate: 12 to 15
Advanced: failure

Kneeling cable pulldown

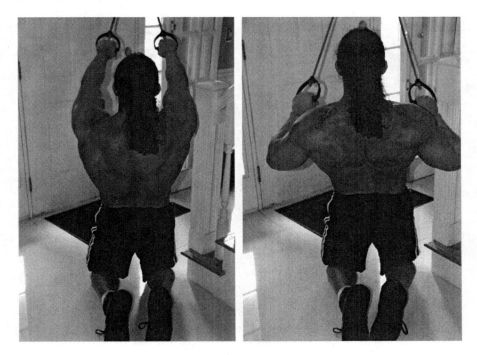

This exercise will benefit the upper and middle portions of your back, along with your biceps

- Attach an exercise band or tubing to the top of a door with a door attachment. Kneel down on the floor and back away from the door to allow tension on the upper back muscles with your arms straight.
- Begin the movement by pulling your arms down, bending at the elbow. Be sure to keep your body upright as you pull down. Focus on your back muscles doing all of the work in pulling the cable down.
- Finish the movement by straightening out your arms, feeling a good stretch in your back muscles.

Number of repetitions:

Beginner: 10 to 12

Intermediate: 12 to 15

Advanced: failure

One-arm dumbbell row

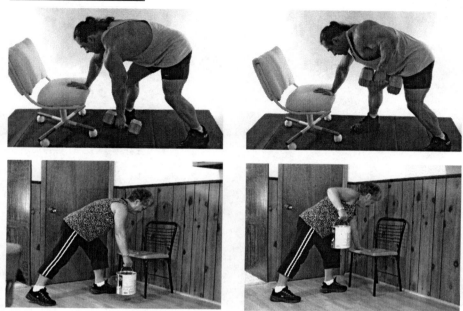

This exercise will benefit the upper and middle portions of your back, along with your biceps

- Kneel with your right knee on a bench or other stable surface. Have your right hand secured on the stable surface, as well. Have your left foot flat on the floor, about a foot out from the bench.
- Grasp one dumbbell in your left hand. You can use a weighted paint can or other household item if dumbbells are not available.
- Begin by bringing your elbow up as far as you can while keeping it as close as possible to your body.
- Focus on squeezing your back muscles, visualizing your arm as merely a hook between your back and the dumbbell.
- Complete all repetitions before switching arms.
- When the dumbbell is in your right hand, your left knee and hand should now be on the bench, with your right foot down flat and vice-versa.

Number of repetitions:

Beginner: 10 to 12

Intermediate: 8 to 10

Advanced: 6 to 8

Dumbbell shrug

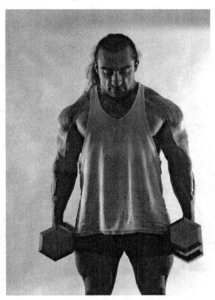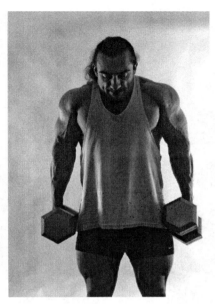

This exercise will benefit your trapezius (upper back muscles connecting to your neck), as well as your upper back, shoulders and forearms.

- Stand with dumbbells in each hand.
- Keep your arms straight down.
- Slightly lower your chin.
- Begin by lifting your shoulders as high as possible, as if trying to touch your ears.
- Focus on squeezing the trapezius muscle at the top before lowering your shoulders to the starting position.

Number of repetitions:
Beginner: 10 to 12
Intermediate: 8 to 12
Advanced: 6 to 10

Reverse-grip cable pulldown

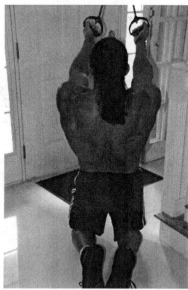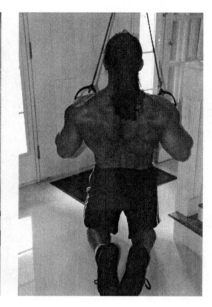

This exercise will benefit the upper and middle portions of your back, along with your biceps

- Attach an exercise band or tubing to the top of the door with door attachment.
- Kneel down on the floor facing the door, and back up away from the door to allow constant tension on the upper back muscles, keeping arms straight.
- Have the palms of your hands facing out when starting.
- Begin the movement by turning your palms inward as you bring your elbows down and back simultaneously.
- Focus on squeezing the back muscles on the way down and slowly return to the starting stretched position.

Number of repetitions:
Beginner: 10 to 12
Intermediate: 12 to 15
Advanced: failure

Bent-over dumbbell row

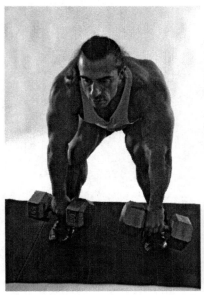 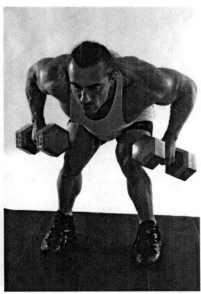

This exercise will benefit the upper and middle portions of your back, along with your biceps

- Bend forward at the knees and hips, keeping your head and chest up. This will help keep an arch in your lower back.
- Start with your arms fully extended, with a maximum stretch in your back.
- Lift the dumbbells up toward your upper abdomen. Focus on your back muscles doing all of the work in lifting the dumbbells. Think of your arms as hooks, just holding the dumbbells.

Number of repetitions:
Beginner: 10 to 12
Intermediate: 8 to 10
Advanced: 6 to 8

Dumbbell upright row

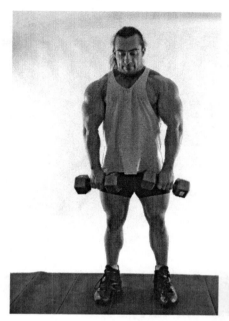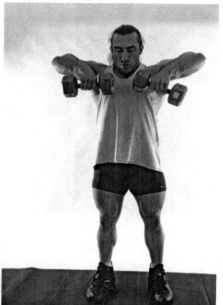

This exercise will benefit your upper back muscles, trapezius, front part of your shoulder, biceps, and forearms.

- Stand with knees slightly bent.
- Keep your chin down as you lift the dumbbells to your chin, leading with the elbows.
- Keep the dumbbells close together and return to the starting position.

Number of repetitions:
Beginner: 10 to 12
Intermediate: 8 to 10
Advanced: 6 to 8

Back extension on Swiss ball

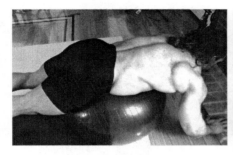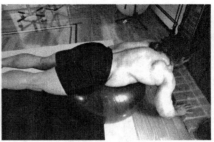

This exercise will primarily benefit your lower back and hamstrings, with some benefit to your abdomen.

- Lay with your stomach on top of the Swiss ball.
- Position yourself so your pelvis is in contact with the ball. Your legs should be straight with feet off the floor. Your hands should be in contact with the floor for balance.
- Begin movement by lifting your legs while squeezing your gluteal muscles. Be sure to keep your legs straight throughout the movement.
- Bring your legs up high enough to get a good squeeze in the lower back and gluteal muscles.
- Slowly return to the starting position.

Number of repetitions:
Beginner: 10 to 12
Intermediate: 12 to 15
Advanced: failure

Dumbbell deadlift

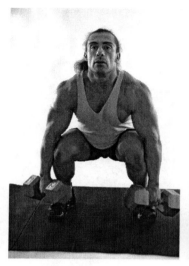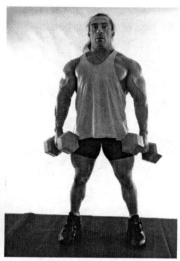

This exercise will benefit your upper back, trapezius, middle back, lower back, shoulders, biceps, forearms, quadriceps, and hamstrings.

- Stand with a dumbbell in each hand.
- Be sure to keep your feet flat on the floor throughout the entire movement. Begin by squatting down, being sure to keep your head and chest up, which will maintain an arch in your lower back.
- Squat down low enough so your thighs are at least parallel to the floor. (Dumbbells should be just shy of coming in contact with the ground.)
- Focus on using your legs to stand up straight, completing the movement.

Number of repetitions:
Beginner: 10 to 12
Intermediate: 8 to 10
Advanced: 6 to 8

LEGS

The leg muscle, one of the largest in the body, includes the front of our thighs (quadriceps), the back of our thighs (hamstrings), and the inner and outer thigh muscles. You can think of our hamstrings as our legs' bicep muscles.

Similar to our biceps, which flex our arms at the elbow, our hamstrings flex our legs at the knee. Conversely, you can think of our quadriceps as the triceps of our legs. Just as the triceps contract with extension of the arm, our quadriceps contract with the extension of the leg. Having strong inner and outer thighs will help with leg strength and balance.

Leg exercises

Wall squats on Swiss ball

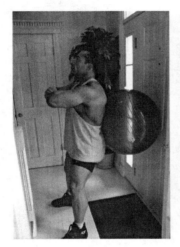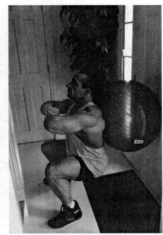

This exercise will primarily benefit your large quadriceps muscles, which make up the front of your thighs.

- Stand with your lower back in contact with an exercise ball against a flat wall.
- Stand with your feet far out in front at shoulder-width apart or slightly narrower.
- Slide down so your knees are at a 90-degree angle.
- Your thighs should be parallel to the floor as you begin to stand up straight.
- At the top of the movement, keep a slight bend in your knees to help maintain constant tension in the quadriceps muscle. (In other words, avoid locking out your knees while standing.)

- Be sure when you are squatting down that your knees never slide forward, beyond your feet. (This would place unnecessary stress to your knees and increase the risk of injury.)

Number of repetitions:

Beginner: 10 to 12

Intermediate: 12 to 15

Advanced: failure

Cable single leg extension

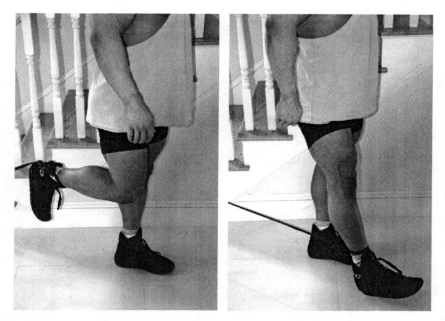

This exercise will primarily benefit your large quadriceps muscles, which make up the front of your thighs.

- Attach an exercise band to a low point, with a loop at the end.
- Place the foot of your "working" leg through the loop, so the band is around your ankle. Elevate your leg so the foot of the "working" leg is off the floor.
- Grab on to a secure object for balance. The knee should be bent at the starting position. Begin the movement by extending the leg straight out.

- Avoid moving the hip. Flexion and extension should occur only at the knee joint.
- Keep the tempo slower when returning to the starting position.
- Complete all repetitions with one leg before moving to the other.

Number of repetitions:

Beginner: 10 to 12

Intermediate: 12 to 15

Advanced: failure

Cable single leg curl

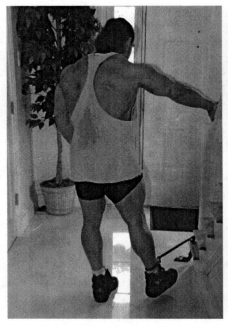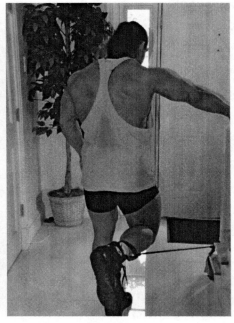

This exercise will primarily benefit your hamstrings, which are in the back of your thigh from just above your calves all the way up to your buttocks.

- Attach an exercise band to a low point, with a loop at the end. Place the foot of your "working" leg through the loop, so the band is around the ankle.
- Elevate your leg so the foot of the "working" leg is off of the floor. Grab on to a secure object for balance. The leg should be straight at the starting position.

- Begin the movement by flexing the knee, as if trying to touch your buttocks with your heel. Focus on squeezing your hamstring.
- Slowly return to the starting position.
- Finish all repetitions with one leg before switching to the other leg.

Number of repetitions:

Beginner: 10 to 12

Intermediate: 12 to 15

Advanced: failure

Cable single leg hip extension

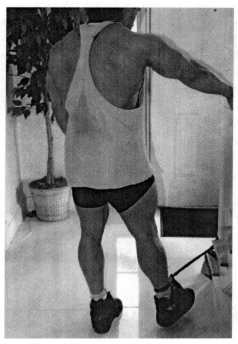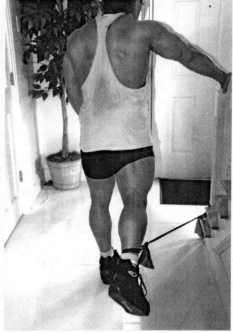

This exercise will benefit your hamstrings and gluteal (buttocks) muscles.

- Attach an exercise band to a low point, with a loop at the end.
- Place the foot of your "working" leg through the loop, so the band is around the ankle. Elevate your leg so the foot of the "working" leg is off the floor.
- Grab on to a secure object for balance. The leg should be straight throughout the movement.

- Start by extending your leg back and out to your side (posterior-laterally). Focus on squeezing the muscles of your hip.
- Slowly return back to the starting position, and complete all repetitions with one leg before turning around and working the other leg.

Number of repetitions:

Beginner: 10 to 12

Intermediate: 12 to 15

Advanced: failure

<u>Dumbbell squat</u>

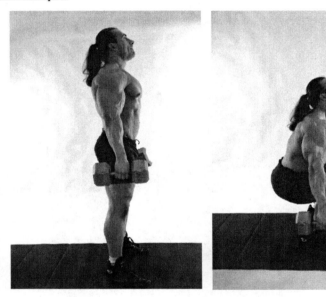

This exercise will benefit nearly all of the muscles from below the waist, primarily focusing on your quadriceps, with involvement of your hamstrings, gluteal muscles and calves.

- Stand with feet shoulder-width apart, holding a dumbbell in each hand (optional), resting at shoulder level or out to your side.
- Keep your head and chest up as you bend your knees until your thighs are parallel to the floor.
- Keep the abdominals tight and maintain weight on your heels, as you stand up straight.

- Avoid locking the knees at the top of the movement. In other words, maintain a slight bend of the knees at the top of the movement, ensuring constant tension on the quadriceps.

Number of repetitions:

Beginner: 10 to 12

Intermediate: 8 to 10

Advanced: 6 to 8

Chair Squat

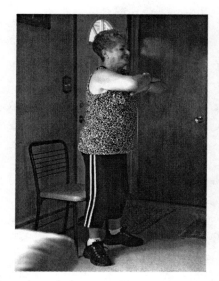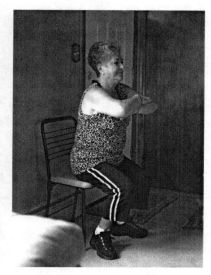

If you have balance problems, squats can be performed using a chair. Simply stand in front of a chair that is positioned against a wall and lower yourself until your buttocks gently touches the chair. Immediately rise and continue to perform the designated sets and repetitions.

Dumbbell split squat

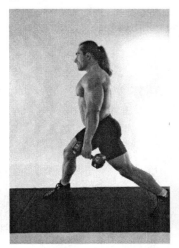 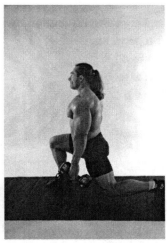

This exercise will benefit nearly all of the muscles from below the waist, primarily focusing on your quadriceps, with involvement of your hamstrings, gluteal muscles and calves.

- Stand with one foot in front, flat on the floor. Back foot should be far back, with only the ball of the back foot in contact with the ground.
- Have a dumbbell in each hand for added resistance.
- Starting with the right leg in front, genuflect, bringing your left knee down as close to the ground as possible without touching.
- Focusing on squeezing the right thigh and buttocks, bring yourself up to a starting position.
- Keep repetitions constant. Avoid resting at the top or bottom of the movement.
- Complete all repetitions with one leg before switching to the other.

Number of repetitions:
Beginner: 10 to 12
Intermediate: 8 to 10
Advanced: 6 to 8

Stiff-leg deadlift

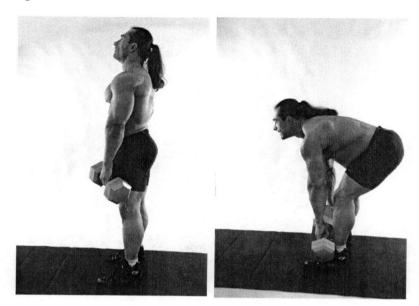

This exercise will primarily work your hamstrings and gluteal muscles.

- Hold a dumbbell in each hand, letting them hang down in front of your thighs. Ensure the dumbbells remain as close to your legs as possible throughout the movement. This will help protect your lower back.
- Keep your legs straight and your head and chest up as you bend forward, achieving a good stretch in your hamstrings.
- Focus on contracting the hamstrings and gluteal muscles as you raise your torso until in-line with your legs.
- Keep the tempo slow, really focusing on standing up straight with your hamstrings and buttocks doing all of the work on getting you up straight. You are NOT initiating the movement with your lower back.

Number of repetitions:

Beginner: 12 to 15

Intermediate: 10 to 12

Advanced: 8 to 12

Single-leg stiff-leg deadlift

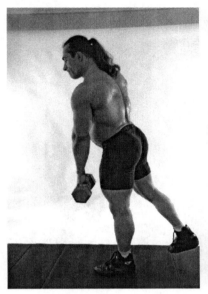 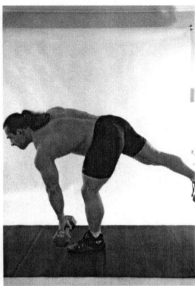

This exercise will primarily benefit your hamstrings and gluteal muscles.
Warning: *This is an advanced-level exercise that should be performed only by those with excellent balance.*

- If starting with your left leg, stand with your left leg straight.
- Hold a dumbbell in your left hand.
- Keep your head and chest up as you bend forward at the waist, allowing your right foot to go back. Go far enough forward to achieve a good stretch in the left hamstring.
- From there, squeeze the left buttocks and hamstring to get your body upright.
- Go down slowly; faster as you get back up, in order to keep the focus on your hamstrings. By lowering your body too rapidly, you increase the chances of losing tension on the hamstrings and placing too much stress on the lower back.
- Complete all repetitions with one leg before moving to the other.

Number of repetitions:
Beginner: 12 to 15
Intermediate: 10 to 12
Advanced: 8 to 12

Lying leg curl on Swiss ball

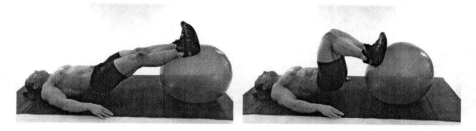

This exercise will primarily benefit your hamstrings and gluteal muscles.

- Lie on the floor with legs straight, and ankles resting on top of Swiss ball.
- Begin the movement by lifting your pelvis up off the floor with your buttocks.
- From there, bend your knees and squeeze your hamstrings and buttocks as you bring your heels as close to your buttocks as possible.
- Slowly return to the starting position.
- Be sure to keep constant tension on your hamstrings throughout the movement.

No. of repetitions:
Beginner: 10 to 12
Intermediate: 12 to 15
Advanced: failure

Sissy squat

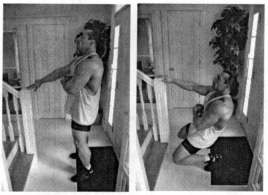

This exercise will primarily benefit your large quadriceps muscles, which make up the front of your thighs, with some involvement of your hamstrings and gluteal muscles.

Warning: *This is a more advanced exercise worth paying close attention to, in order to minimize risk of knee injury.*

- Stand with feet about shoulder-width apart or even slightly more narrow.
- Hold onto a stable surface like a pole for balance.
- Keep your body upright as you squat down, lifting your heels off the ground so that only the balls of your feet are in contact with the ground. Squat down to a point where your buttocks is almost touching your heels.
- At this point, you will flex your quadriceps, allowing yourself to rise to the starting position. Heels now return to the ground.
- Be sure to go down slowly, in about three to four seconds. Rise more rapidly, in about one second.
- Focus on feeling a good stretch in your quadriceps as you go down.
- For added resistance, hold a dumbbell in your free hand against your chest.

Number of repetitions:
Beginner: 10 to 12
Intermediate: 12 to 15
Advanced: failure

Dumbbell walking lunge

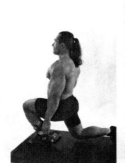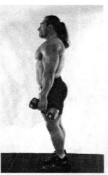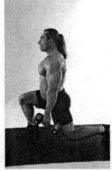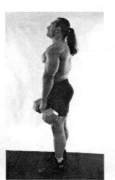

This exercise will benefit nearly all of the muscles below the waist, primarily focusing on your quadriceps, with involvement of your hamstrings, gluteal muscles and calves.

- Stand with a dumbbell in each hand.
- If starting with your left leg, take a big step with your left leg forward.

- From there, genuflect, bringing your right knee as close to the floor as possible without touching. Be sure your left knee doesn't travel past your left toes, to prevent excessive stress on the knee.
- The lunge continues by bringing your right knee back up, flexing the left thigh and gluteal muscles hard.
- You will then move on by taking a giant step with the right leg, followed by bringing your left knee down low without touching the floor.
- Continue the sequence in the same manner.

Number of repetitions:

Beginner: 10 to 12

Intermediate: 8 to 12

Advanced: failure

Cable hip adduction

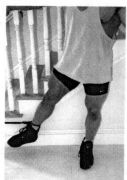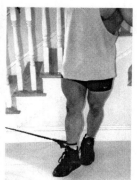

This exercise will benefit your inner thigh area.

- Attach an exercise band to a low point with a loop at the end.
- Place the foot of your "working" leg through the loop, so the band is around your ankle. Elevate your leg so the foot of the "working" leg is off the floor. Grab onto a secure object for balance. The leg should be straight throughout the movement.
- If starting with the left leg, stand far enough away from the cable attachment site so you feel resistance against the left inner thigh. Your left shoulder is pointed in the direction of the attachment site.
- Begin the movement by moving your foot in the direction toward the midline of your body, to a point of maximal contraction of the left inner thigh.

- Slowly return to the starting position.
- Maintain constant tension on the inner thighs.
- Complete all repetitions with one leg before switching sides.

Number of repetitions:
Beginner: 10 to 12
Intermediate: 12 to 15
Advanced: failure

<u>Cable hip abduction</u>

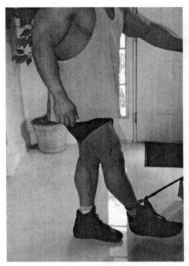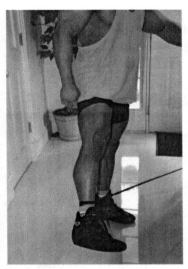

This exercise will benefit your outer thigh and hip region.

- Setup is the same for hip adduction. Where it differs is if starting with the left leg, your right shoulder should be pointed in the direction of the attachment site. Also, you should be standing far enough away from the attachment site so enough tension is on the left outer thigh/hip area at rest.
- Begin the movement by extending the left leg out to the left.
- Slowly return to the starting position.
- Complete all repetitions with one leg before moving to the other.

Number of repetitions:
Beginner: 10 to 12
Intermediate: 12 to 15
Advanced: failure

Calves

The calves are the muscles at the back of the lower legs. They are made up of two muscles – the gastrocnemius and soleus. Both of these muscles function in flexing the foot. When you stand up on the balls of your feet, you are working these muscles. The gastrocnemius is more of an explosive muscle, engaged with activities such as jumping, sprinting and explosively flexing your foot. The soleus is a larger and deeper portion of the muscle that connects into the Achilles tendon and inserts into the heel bone. It is engaged more with calf exercises in which you are either seated or have a bend in the knees.

The calves are a stubborn muscle group and need to be worked more frequently with shorter rest periods between sets. The stubbornness of this muscle group may have to do with the fact that the muscle is constantly being stimulated when we walk on our feet all day. As a result, it takes a little extra effort to get these muscles to respond and grow the way we'd like them to. They respond well to heavy weights and high repetitions. I usually keep rest periods to no more than 60 seconds for this particular muscle group.

Calf Exercises

<u>Standing calf raise</u>

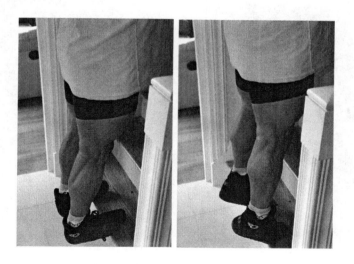

This exercise will primarily benefit your gastrocnemius muscles.

- Stand on a stable board or step so that only the balls of your feet are on the step.
- Knees should be slightly bent.
- Lower your heels as far as comfortably possible for a maximum stretch and rise up on your toes as high as possible.
- Each repetition should consist of two contractions. When you first rise up on the balls of your feet as high as possible, you will find that you can still get higher up by squeezing a second time here. So when counting repetitions, you should be counting "one, two; one, two; one, two;" etc.
- Rest period should be less than 60 seconds, as the calf muscles recover fairly quickly between sets.

Number of repetitions:

Beginner: 10 to 12

Intermediate: 12 to 15

Advanced: failure

Single calf raise on step

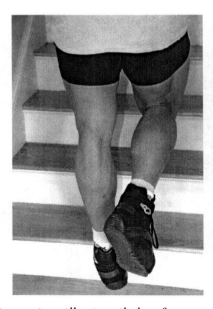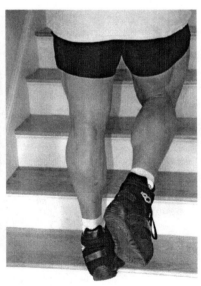

This exercise will primarily benefit your gastrocnemius muscles. Bending your knees will recruit more of the soleus muscle.

- Stand with the ball of one foot on a step. Hold one dumbbell for added resistance (optional) and grab a stable object with the other hand for balance.
- Begin the movement by lowering the heel of your working leg as far as possible for a maximum stretch.
- Focus on squeezing your calf muscle as you stand tall on your toes. Perform the movement in the same fashion as the standing calf raise.
- Complete all repetitions with one leg before switching to the other.
- Rest period should be less than 60 seconds, as the calf muscles recover fairly quickly between sets.

Number of repetitions:

Beginner: 10 to 12

Intermediate: 12 to 15

Advanced: failure

Abdominal Muscles

There are several muscles that make up the abdomen. The rectus abdominis is the main skeletal muscle of the belly. Its main function is to flex the spine. You can think of it as the opposite of the muscles of the lower back, which work to extend and stabilize the spine. The external obliques are the muscles along each side of the rectus abdominis. These muscles flex and rotate the spine. The intercostals are another set of abdominal muscles, which occupy the space between the ribs. Their main function is to lift up the ribs and bring them together.

Although I have listed below several exercises to target the abdominal muscles, keep in mind that they are being worked with the majority of the exercises we perform – especially those performed on a Swiss ball. This is mainly because these are some of our major stabilizer muscles, which work to keep us balanced on this unstable ball.

Abdominal Exercises

Abdominal crunch on
Swiss ball (beginner)

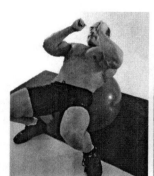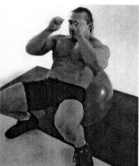

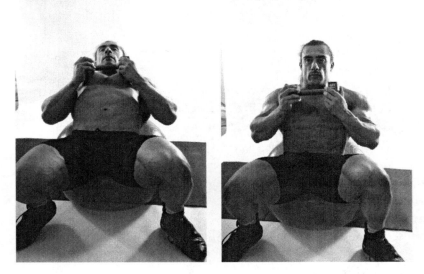

This exercise will benefit your core stabilizer muscles – abdominals, obliques and lower back muscles

- Sit on a Swiss ball. Hold onto a stable object for support if necessary.
- Begin by slowly leaning back to a comfortable stretch.
- Exhale as you crunch forward, sitting up and flexing your abdomen.
- Complete all repetitions in a slow, controlled fashion.
- Use a dumbbell for added resistance if you prefer.

Number of repetitions:

Beginner: 8 to 12

Intermediate: 12 to 15

Advanced: failure

V-ups on floor

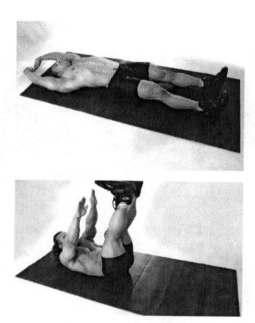

This exercise will benefit your abdominals and obliques.

- Lie flat on the floor with feet together and legs out straight. Arms should be straight back with back of hands on floor.
- Begin movement by crunching abdomen as you raise your feet and arms simultaneously, as if trying to touch your shins.
- Focus on squeezing your abdominal muscles as you crunch.
- Exhale as you crunch and inhale as you return to starting position.

Number of repetitions:

Beginner: 8 to 12

Intermediate: 12 to 15

Advanced: failure

<u>Lying leg raise on Swiss ball</u>

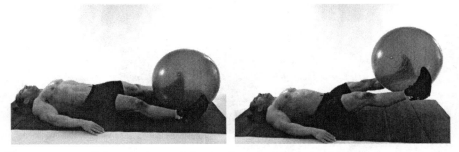

This exercise will benefit your abdominals and obliques, with greater emphasis on your lower abdominals.

- Lie flat on the floor with legs straight. Keep hands flat on the floor and close to your side. Position a Swiss ball between your feet.
- Keeping your legs straight, slowly lift the ball with your feet. Exhale as you lift the ball. Inhale as you lower the ball to the lowest point without touching the floor.
- Contrary to other exercises, you will perform the rising and lowering phases in the same tempo – over four seconds. Keep the repetitions slow and continuous.

Number of repetitions:
Beginner: 8 to 12
Intermediate: 12 to 15
Advanced: failure

Shoulders

The shoulder is a three-headed muscle that makes up your upper arm, originating from your scapula and clavicle. The largest and strongest of the three heads is the front deltoid. Its main function is to press up. The second-largest is the side deltoid. It is engaged when we lift our arms out to our sides. The smallest and usually weakest of the three heads is the rear deltoid. It is engaged when pulling back. If you were to do a row with the elbows up high toward your neck, this muscle group would be targeted.

Shoulder Exercises

<u>Arnold Press</u>

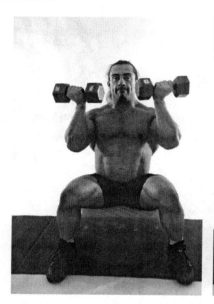 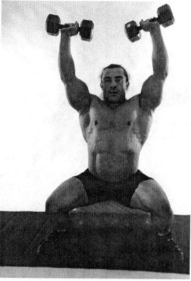

Due to the twisting motion involved, this press will benefit the front, side and rear heads of the shoulder muscle. The core stabilizer muscles will also receive some benefit.

- Sit on a Swiss ball with a dumbbell in each hand.
- Starting position is palms facing you with dumbbells at shoulder level. It looks like the finishing position of a dumbbell biceps curl.
- Begin by pressing the dumbbells overhead, simultaneously rotating the palms outward.
- Immediately lower the weight while rotating the wrists so palms face inward with dumbbells at shoulder level.
- Dumbbells must always be positioned directly above the elbows and never lowered below shoulder level.

Number of repetitions:

Beginner: 10 to 12

Intermediate: 8 to 10

Advanced: 6 to 8

Bent-over dumbbell rear lateral raise

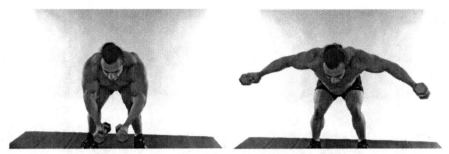

This exercise will mainly benefit the rear head of your shoulders, with some recruitment of your triceps.

- Bend forward at the knees and hips with chest up and head neutral with your spine. Keep your neck relaxed throughout the motion.
- Have dumbbells out in front and close to your body.
- Keep elbows slightly bent as you drive the dumbbells out to the side and back.
- Keep the dumbbells in line with your shoulders. You are forming an arc or half-circle with your arms. It's as if you were performing a reverse bear hug or the opposite motion of the cable chest fly.

Number of repetitions:
Beginner: 12 to 15
Intermediate: 10 to 12
Advanced: 8 to 12

One-arm external rotation

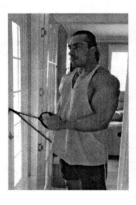
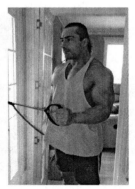

This exercise will benefit the side head of your shoulder, with emphasis to your rotator cuff muscles (small stabilizer muscles of your shoulder joint). This is one exercise where you need not use heavy resistance. The primary objective is to target your small (weak) stabilizer muscles. With too heavy a resistance, the rotator cuff muscles will not be activated. Rather, pick a resistance you can handle for a good 12 to 15 repetitions.

- Stand with an exercise band tied to a secure bar at about waistline, with your working arm across your body and grabbing the band.
- Begin by rotating your arm away from your torso, keeping your upper arm against your body.
- Visualize holding a towel up to your body with your elbow, as you externally rotate the arm.
- Complete all repetitions with one arm before switching arms.

Number of repetitions:
Beginner: 12 to 15
Intermediate: 12 to 15
Advanced: 12 to 15

Dumbbell front lateral raise

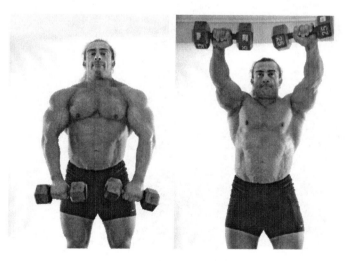

This exercise will benefit the front head of your shoulder, as well as your biceps and forearms.

- Keep knees slightly bent, with arms out in front.
- Keep arms straight with elbows locked as you raise dumbbells to eye level. If you don't have access to dumbbells, use weighted paint cans or other household items.
- Slowly return to the starting position.

Number of repetitions:

Beginner: 10 to 12

Intermediate: 8 to 10

Advanced: 6 to 10

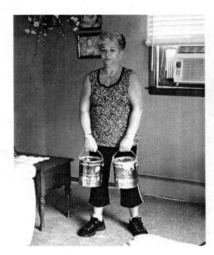 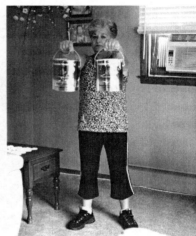

Side dumbbell lateral raise

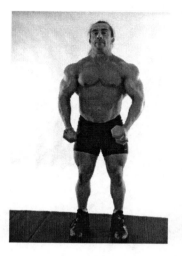

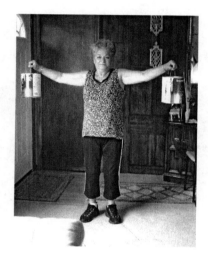

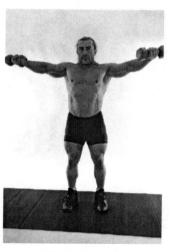

This exercise will benefit the side head of your shoulder.

- Stand with knees slightly bent and dumbbells in hand hanging out to your sides. Use weighted paint cans or other household items if dumbbells are unavailable. Maintain a bend in the elbows of about 30 degrees.
- Raise dumbbells and elbows level with the shoulders, rotating to palms-down at the beginning of the motion. In other words, turn your wrists as if pouring pitchers of water. Be sure to lead the motion with the elbows.
- Slowly return to the starting position.

Number of repetitions:
Beginner: 10 to 12
Intermediate: 8 to 10
Advanced: 6 to 10

<u>One-arm dumbbell side lateral raise</u>

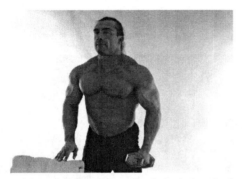 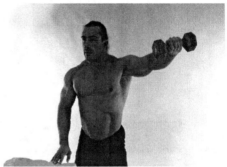

This exercise will benefit the side head of your shoulder.

- Same sequence as the dumbbell side lateral raise except you're now working with one arm at a time.
- The resting arm should hold onto a stable object for balance and stabilization.

Number of repetitions:
Beginner: 10 to 12
Intermediate: 8 to 10
Advanced: 6 to 10

Triceps

The triceps is the muscle that makes up the back of our upper arm. It actually composes about 60% of our arm. Men will sometimes ask me what to do to get big arms. They are under the misconception that you need to be doing more bicep curls to get these arms to grow. They are usually quite surprised when I tell them to work their triceps more. I inform them that the bicep muscle is simply the "icing on the cake," or the "cherry on top."

Women tend to be equally surprised after asking me what the best exercises are to lose the flab on the back of the upper arm. To really get to the meat of the arm, you need to be working the triceps.

Triceps got its name from the fact that there are three heads to the muscle. The main function of this muscle is to straighten out the arm, and it is involved with pressing movements.

Triceps Exercises

<u>Close-grip pushup on counter</u>

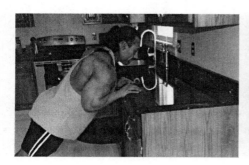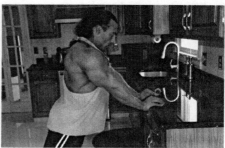

This exercise will primarily benefit your triceps, as well as your chest and front of your shoulders.

- Stand several feet away from a counter or other stable surface.
- Stand on the balls of your feet and keep the abs tight as you place your hands on the counter about one foot apart. Be sure to keep elbows fixed at your sides.
- Lower your chest toward the counter and press up, focusing on the triceps muscles doing all of the work in pressing your body up.
- Go slower in the lowering (stretching) phase than in pressing.

Number of repetitions:
Beginner: 10 to 12
Intermediate: 12 to 15
Advanced: failure

Dumbbell close-grip press on Swiss ball
Please note: You can purchase a Swiss ball from most sports stores as well as the fitness section of a department store

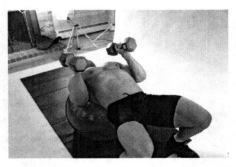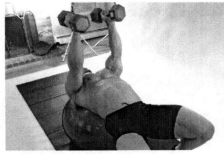

This exercise will primarily benefit your triceps, as well as your chest and front of your shoulders. Being that this exercise is performed on a Swiss ball, your core stabilizer muscles will also benefit.

- Sit on a Swiss with a dumbbell in each hand.
- Walk your feet forward as you slide back on the ball to a starting position with your upper back and neck supported against the ball. This should be a relatively comfortable position.
- Begin the movement by slowly pressing the dumbbells up to an end position of having your arms straight with a slight bend in the elbows, ensuring constant tension on the chest muscles.
- Unlike the dumbbell chest press on Swiss ball, your elbows must be kept as close to your body as possible. Keep your palms facing each other throughout the movement.
- Slowly return the dumbbells to the starting position, obtaining a comfortable stretch.

Number of repetitions:
Beginner: 10 to 12
Intermediate: 8 to 10
Advanced: 6 to 10

One-arm triceps extension

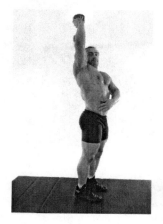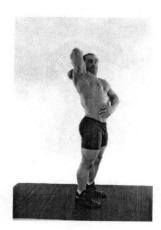

This exercise will benefit your triceps.

- Stand grabbing one end of a dumbbell or exercise band overhead with your working arm. Your other hand should be behind your back with your resting arm.
- The starting position is with your working arm fully bent at the elbow, keeping your elbow as close to your head as possible.
- To complete the movement, straighten out your working arm to full extension, keeping your elbow as close to your head as possible. Complete all repetitions with one arm before switching to the other.

Number of repetitions:

Beginner: 10 to 12

Intermediate: 8 to 10

Advanced: 6 to 10

One-arm dumbbell triceps kickback

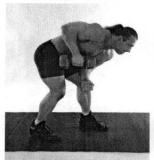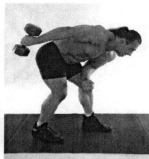

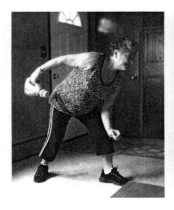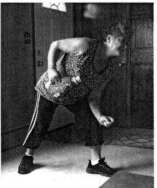

This exercise will benefit your triceps.

- Bend forward, keeping the elbow of the arm with the dumbbell as close to your body as possible. You can use a detergent bottle or other weighted household item if a dumbbell is unavailable.
- Begin the movement with your arm flexed, and simply extend the lower arm back, keeping the elbow fixed to your side.
- Pause at the top of the movement for one second before returning the weight to the starting position.
- Complete all repetitions with one arm before switching to the other.

Number of repetitions:

Beginner: 10 to 12

Intermediate: 8 to 10

Advanced: 6 to 10

Reverse-grip triceps extension

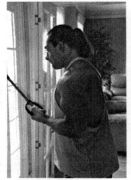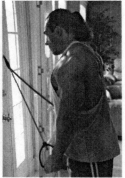

This exercise will benefit your triceps

- Stand with an exercise band tied to a secure bar no lower than the level of your midline.
- Grasp the band in one arm, with your palm facing up. Keep your elbow flexed and as close to your body as possible. Your nonworking arm should hold onto a bar or other stable surface for maximum stability.
- Complete the contraction by straightening out the arm and holding for a one-second pause, before returning to the flexed, starting position.
- Complete all repetitions with one arm before switching to the other.

Number of repetitions:
Beginner: 10 to 12
Intermediate: 8 to 10
Advanced: 6 to 10

Close-grip pushup

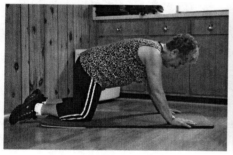 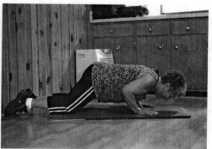

This exercise will primarily benefit your triceps, as well as your chest and front of your shoulders.

- Begin by getting down on all four limbs, keeping arms and legs straight. Balls of your feet should be in contact with the floor. If you lack the strength to handle push-ups in this position, you could perform them with knees in contact with the floor. As you get stronger, you can progress to the traditional form with the balls of your feet planted on the floor.
- Distance between your hands should be about one foot. Be sure to keep your elbows as close to your body as possible
- Start the motion by lowering your chest towards the floor, bending the elbows.

- Just before touching the floor with your chest, press up, straightening out your arms as you come up. The lowering phase should be done slower than the rising phase.

Number of repetitions:

Beginner: 10 to 12

Intermediate: 12 to 15 repetitions to failure

Advanced: failure

<u>Lying triceps extension on Swiss ball</u>

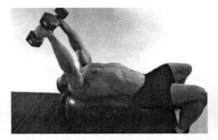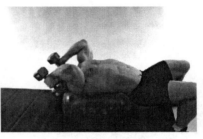

This exercise will benefit your triceps, as well as your core stabilizer muscles.

- Start by sitting on a Swiss ball and walk forward as you lean back to a point where your head and upper back are in contact with the Swiss ball.
- Have a dumbbell in each hand and raise your arms straight up.
- Slowly lower the dumbbells toward the back of your head, bending at the elbows. Be sure to keep your elbows in, toward your head and ears.
- Complete the movement by straightening out your arms.

Number of repetitions:

Beginner: 10 to 12

Intermediate: 8 to 10

Advanced: 6 to 10

Biceps

The biceps muscle is a two-headed muscle that makes up the front of the upper arm. You can think of it as the opposite of the triceps muscle. Its major function is to flex the arm at the elbow. It is also involved in pulling exercises. Your brachioradialis muscle works synergistically with your biceps, flexing your forearm at your elbow. Certain exercises below will place extra emphasis on your brachioradialis.

Biceps Exercises

Dumbbell biceps curl

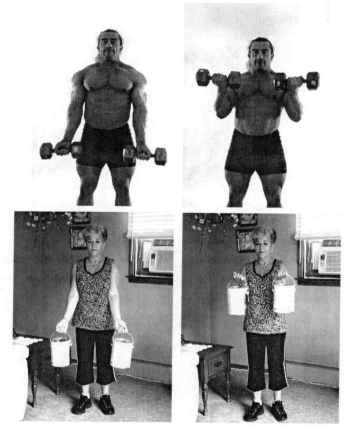

This exercise will mainly benefit your biceps muscles.

- Stand with your knees slightly bent.
- Keep your arms out in front with your elbows fixed to your sides.
- Slowly curl arms toward your shoulders, focusing on squeezing the biceps with each contraction. Use weighted paint cans or other household items if dumbbells are not available.

Number of repetitions:

Beginner: 10 to 12

Intermediate: 8 to 10

Advanced: 6 to 8

Dumbbell hammer curl

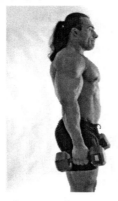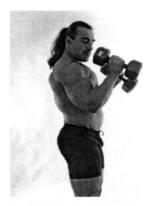

This exercise will primarily target your brachioradialis and forearm muscles. Because it is a smaller component of your biceps, the brachioradialis tends to be weaker. As a result, use lighter weights than you would select for a traditional biceps curl.

- Stand with your knees slightly bent.
- Keep your hands in a thumbs-up position, so dumbbells stay vertical.
- Flex your biceps as you curl your arms toward your shoulders.

Number of repetitions:

Beginner: 10 to 12

Intermediate: 10 to 12

Advanced: 8 to12

Seated one-arm dumbbell concentration curl

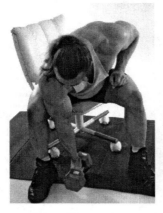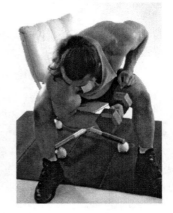

This exercise will benefit your biceps muscles.

- Sit on the corner of a bench or secure seat.
- If beginning with your left arm, rest your left triceps against your left inner thigh. Place your right hand on top of your right thigh for balance.
- Begin by curling the weight up, strictly focusing on squeezing your biceps muscle. Slowly return the weight to the starting position.
- Complete all repetitions with one arm before switching to the other.

Number of repetitions:

Beginner: 10 to 12

Intermediate: 8 to 10

Advanced: 6 to 8

Reverse dumbbell curl

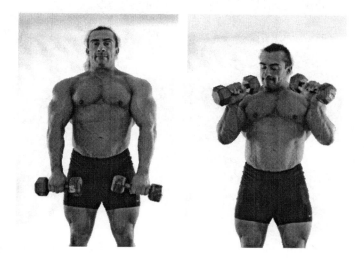

This exercise will primarily target your brachioradialis and forearm muscles. Because it is a smaller component of your biceps, the brachioradialis tends to be weaker. As a result, use lighter weights than you would select for a traditional biceps curl.

- Stand with your knees slightly bent.
- Hold the dumbbells with your palms facing you. Keep your arms out in front with your elbows fixed to your sides.
- Slowly curl your arms toward your shoulders and slowly return to the starting position. Avoid flexing or extending your wrists while

performing the movement. Flexion and extension occur only at the elbow joint.

Number of repetitions:

Beginner: 10 to 12

Intermediate: 10 to 12

Advanced: 8 to12

One-arm dumbbell curl on Swiss ball

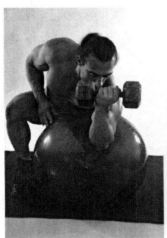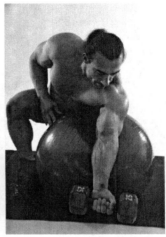

This exercise will benefit your biceps muscles.

Warning: *This is an advanced exercise and should be performed only by those familiar with the Swiss ball. Keep weight light to begin with, as your surface will feel unsteady, increasing your risk of injury.*

- Kneel with a Swiss ball in front of you. If starting with the left arm, rest your left triceps on top of the ball, with a dumbbell in-hand.
- Slowly lower the dumbbell, allowing your arm to almost completely straighten.
- Without resting in the bottom position, squeeze your biceps as you curl the dumbbell up. Keep repetitions continuous, without resting at the top or bottom.
- Keep in mind that by using the Swiss ball, you will not be on a stable surface, which makes the movement more challenging. Thus, you will probably not be able to go as heavy in weight, compared with a traditional dumbbell curl.

- Complete all repetitions with one arm before switching to the other.

Number of repetitions:
Beginner: 10 to 12
Intermediate: 10 to 12
Advanced: 8 to12

Standing alternate dumbbell curl

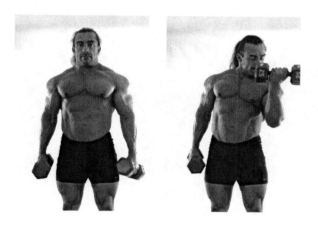

This exercise will benefit your biceps muscles.

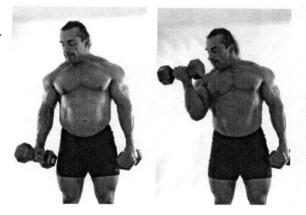

- Stand with a dumbbell in each hand. Keep arms out in front of your body with elbows as close to your sides as possible.

- Begin by flexing the biceps of one arm as you curl the dumbbell up. As you lower the dumbbell down slowly to the starting position, you will begin the same motion with the opposite arm.
- Complete all repetitions with each arm. In other words, if 12 repetitions is your goal, complete 12 repetitions with the left arm and 12 with the right arm for a total of 24 repetitions.
- Lower the dumbbell more slowly than curling it up.
- Be sure to avoid rocking your back.

Number of repetitions:

Beginner: 10 to 12

Intermediate: 8 to 10

Advanced: 6 to 8

Chapter 8

Stretching

The purpose of this chapter is to guide you in putting together a good stretching program. You will learn stretches focusing on the major muscle groups.

A good stretching program should be done at least three times a week, holding each stretch for 10-30 seconds, and repeating three to four times. An ideal time to stretch would be when the body temperature is increased, such as after aerobic or resistance training. Keep in mind that the following stretches are meant to serve as a guide.

You don't have to do every stretch listed here during each session. However, I would include hamstring and lower back stretches with every session, as these muscles tend to tighten quite frequently. Including stretches for the specific muscles you've trained that day would also be wise. For example, if you had worked out your chest and back muscles today, you might complete the workout by stretching the chest, back and hamstrings.

<u>Lower Back Stretches</u>

Knees to Chest

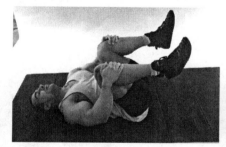 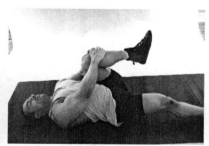

This stretch will loosen the muscles of your lower back and hamstrings.

- Lie flat on the floor or exercise mat with legs straight.
- Slowly bend both knees and bring them as close to your chest as possible, to a point of mild discomfort.
- Keep breathing slowly as you hold the stretch for 10-30 seconds.

- Slowly straighten your legs and rest them on the floor before completing another repetition.
- You can modify the stretch by bringing one knee to the chest at a time. Just remember to keep the other leg straight on the floor.

Hamstring/Low Back Stretch

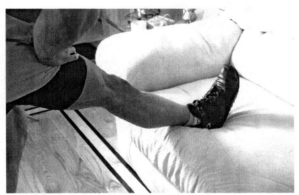

This stretch will loosen the muscles of your lower back and hamstrings.

- Place one ankle on a stable support, such as a bench.
- Keep your other leg straight as you bend forward along the raised leg. Take hold of it as far down as possible.
- Pull gently to get the maximum stretch in the hamstrings.
- Hold for 10-30 seconds, relax, and repeat with the other leg.

Feet-Apart Seated Forward Bends

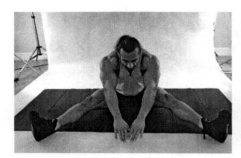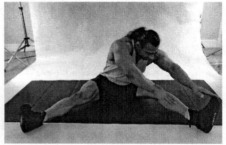

This stretch will loosen the muscles of your lower back, hamstrings, and inner thighs.

- Sit on the floor with your legs straight and wide apart.

- Bend forward and touch the floor with your hands as far in front of you as possible.
- Hold this position for several seconds and then bring your hands over to one leg and grasp it as far down as possible, whether it be your knee, calf, ankle or foot.
- Gently pull to get a full stretch in the hamstring and lower back.
- Hold this position for 10-30 seconds. Then bring your hands over to the other leg and repeat.

Seated Inner Thigh Stretch
This stretch will loosen the muscles of your inner thighs.

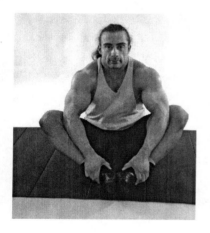

- Sit on the floor and position your legs so the soles of your feet are touching one another. Take hold of your feet and pull them as close to your groin as possible.
- Relax your legs and use your elbows to drop your knees toward the floor, feeling a good stretch in the inner thigh muscles.
- Hold for 10-30 seconds, relax, and repeat for 3-4 total sets.

Seated Hip Stretch
This stretch will loosen your hip and outer thigh muscles.

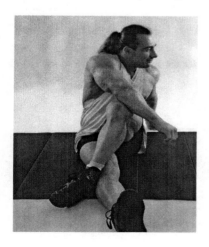

- Begin by sitting on the floor with legs extended in front of you.
- Bring your left knee up and cross your legs so your left foot is placed over your right. Twist around so your right elbow rests on the outside of the left knee.
- Place your left hand on the floor behind you and continue twisting to the left.
- Hold for 10-30 seconds.

- Lower your left knee down and bring your right leg over the left, with right knee up, and repeat the stretch to the opposite side.

Calf Stretch with Leg Back
This stretch will loosen your calf muscles.

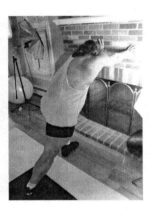

- Lean forward with your hands resting against a stable object (i.e. wall, banister, etc.) with one leg bent forward and the other leg straight back.
- With your leg positioned straight back, bring this leg back as far as possible, being sure to keep the heel of your back foot flat on the floor. You should feel a gentle pull in the calf muscle of your back leg.
- Hold for 10-30 seconds; then repeat with the other leg.

Standing Calf Stretch on Wall
This stretch will loosen your calf muscles.

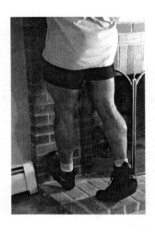

- Find the edge of a wall you can hold for balance and place as much of the bottom of one foot against this wall as you can.
- Thrust your hips forward so your thighs are nearly touching the wall. Be sure to keep the ball of that one foot firmly against the wall. You should feel a gentle pull on that calf muscle.
- Hold for 10-30 seconds; then repeat with the other leg.

Quadriceps Stretch
This stretch will loosen your quadriceps muscles.

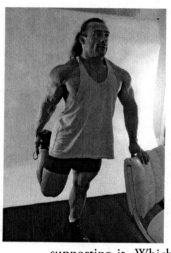

- Stand while holding onto a stable object for balance.
- Grasp your right foot with your right hand and bring your right heel back as close to your right gluteal muscle (butt cheek) as possible. You should feel a stretch at the front of your right thigh.
- Hold for 10-30 seconds; then repeat with the opposite leg.
- For those who have difficulty grasping their foot, place your foot on a chair and lean forward. A better handle on the foot may be achieved with the chair

supporting it. Whichever method you choose, be sure to hold onto a stable object for balance.

Oblique Stretch
This stretch will loosen the obliques as well as other muscles along the sides of the torso.

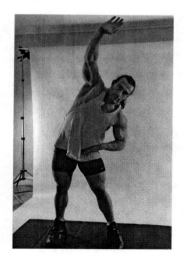

- Begin by standing upright with your feet slightly wider than shoulder-width apart.
- Raise your right arm over your head and slowly bend to the left. Allow your left hand to slide down your thigh, without actually touching it.
- Bend far enough to the side to allow a good stretch to your right side.
- Hold this position for 10-30 seconds.
- Return to the starting position and repeat to the other side.

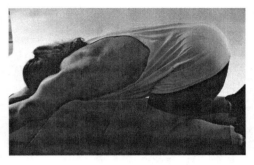

Kneeling Back Stretch
This stretch will help loosen your upper and middle back.

- Begin by getting down on your hands and knees.
- Keeping your knees fixed on the floor or mat, start "walking" your hands forward, to a point where your arms are fully extended, and you feel a maximum stretch in the middle and upper back area.
- Hold for 10-30 seconds.
- Relax and repeat for 3-4 total sets.

Alternate Back Stretch
This stretch will help loosen your upper and middle back, emphasizing each side individually.

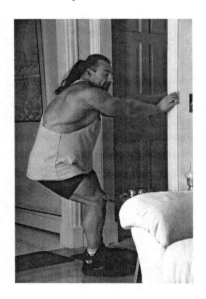

- Find a sturdy pole or banister to grab onto with both hands.
- Start with hips forward and close to the object, then lean back so your arms are fully extended and you reach a maximum stretch in the middle to upper back area.
- To increase the stretch, focus on leaning to one side by relaxing the hip of the same side. For example, if emphasizing the left side of the back, relax your left hip as you straighten the left arm and lean to the left.
- Hold for 10-30 seconds and switch sides for another 10-30 seconds.
- Repeat for a total of 3-4 sets.

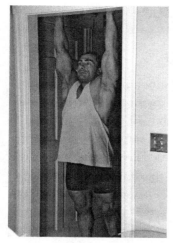

Hanging Back Stretch
This stretch is used to effectively stretch the upper and middle back, relieve tension from the lower back, and help strengthen your forearms.

- Begin by grabbing a chinning bar or an equivalent object, such as a sturdy door frame or heavy-duty spring-type curtain rod at the top of a doorway.
- Hands should be positioned at shoulder-width apart, or slightly narrower.
- Hang on the bar so your feet are off of the floor with arms completely straight.
- Hold for 10-30 seconds.
- Relax and repeat for a total of 3-4 sets.
- To strengthen the forearms in particular, remain in the hanging position as long as possible, trying to beat your previous time with each set.

Chest Stretch
This stretch will help loosen your chest muscles.

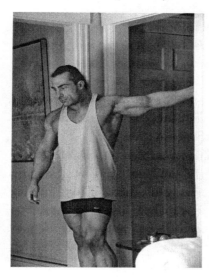

- Place the palm of your left hand on the edge of a wall, with your thumb up, and positioned at eye-level.
- Maintain a slight bend in your left elbow and turn your body to the right.
- Keep turning your feet as far to the right as necessary to give a good stretch to the left chest muscle.
- Hold for 10-30 seconds, relax, then switch to the other side (right hand now on the edge of the wall).

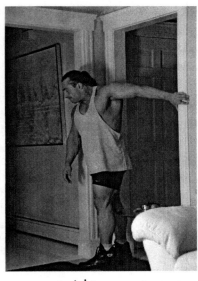

Biceps Stretch
This stretch will help loosen your biceps muscles.

- The positioning for this stretch is similar to the chest stretch, where the palm of your left hand is planted on the edge of a wall.
- The difference is that instead of having your thumb up at eye-level, you will position the hand at neck-level with the thumb down. Another difference: instead of having a slight bend in your left elbow, your left arm will be kept straight, as you turn your feet and upper body to the right.

- ***Warning:*** Be sure to go slowly with this stretch, in particular. The gentle pull you feel can become quite intense with a small turn to the right.
- Hold the stretch for 10-30 seconds; relax, and switch to the opposite arm.

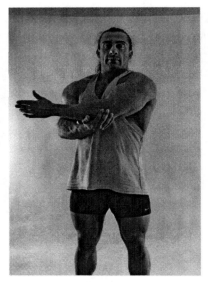

Side Shoulder Stretch
This stretch will help loosen the front and lateral heads of the shoulders.

- Begin by standing up straight, maintaining a slight bend in your left elbow.
- Grab your left elbow with your right hand and bring your left arm across your chest, slowly pushing the left elbow into your chest. You should feel a good stretch to your front and side heads of the left shoulder.
- Hold for 10-30 seconds; relax, and switch to the other arm.

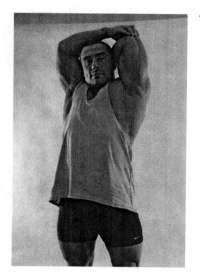

Triceps Stretch
This stretch will help loosen your triceps muscles.

- Stand straight with your left arm bent overhead, as if reaching to scratch your back.
- Grab your left elbow with your right hand and try bringing your elbow back and down as much as possible. You should feel a good stretch in the back of your upper left arm (triceps).
- For an even greater stretch, extend your head back, which should pull your left forearm back and enhance the triceps stretch.
- Hold for 10-30 seconds; relax, and switch to the opposite arm.

Trapezius Stretch

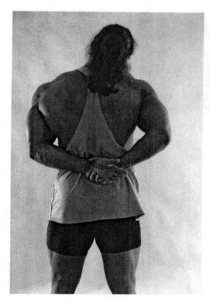
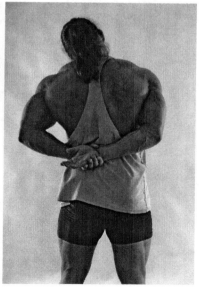

This stretch will loosen your trapezius muscles, going from your upper back to your neck region.

- Stand straight and position your hands behind you.
- Grasp your left wrist with your right hand.
- Using your right hand, pull your wrist down and to the right. At the same time, bring your right ear towards your right shoulder. This will stretch your left upper trapezius muscle.
- Hold this stretch for 10-30 seconds; relax, and switch to the opposite side. Here, you will now grasp your right wrist with your left hand, bringing it down and to the left. Simultaneously, you will bring your left ear towards your left shoulder.
- Hold for 10-30 seconds, and complete 3-4 sets each side.

Neck Stretch

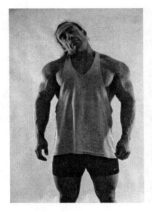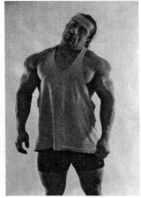

This stretch will help loosen your neck muscles.

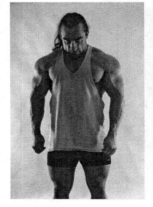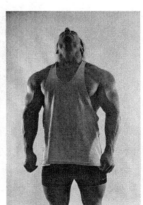

- This is a simple stretch that can be performed either standing or seated. You can start by bringing your left ear toward your left shoulder.
- Hold for 10-30 seconds, and repeat to the opposite side.
- Next, bring your chin towards your chest and hold for 10-30 seconds.
- Finish the routine by trying to touch your upper back with the back of your head.
- Hold each stretch for 10-30 seconds, and repeat each side for a total of 3-4 sets.

Chapter 9

Sample Workouts

I can usually spot new exercisers in my gym. They are walking around lost, overwhelmed by the number of various machines. Not only are they unsure what body part each of these machines will work and how they work, they don't have a plan. It usually isn't long before these new exercisers give up or just focus on aerobics, which tend to be easier to understand. This chapter will provide you with a plan so that you will have the confidence and understanding of how to exercise at home or at your local gym.

Whether you are new to exercise or are just looking for a tweak in your routine, this chapter will provide useful examples. Keep in mind that these are merely samples and you can adjust these exercises to your particular liking. You can change the order of the exercises, the number of sets, the repetitions, and the training days as you see fit.

Beginner Home Workout*

Aerobics can be performed three to seven days per week for 30 to 60 minutes. Alternatively, you can do three 10-minute sessions of aerobics spread throughout the day if a continuous 30-minute session in not yet possible.

If aerobics are done on the same day as resistance training, either perform the aerobics immediately after weight training or pick another time of day to do it. With the exception of five to 10 minutes of aerobics as a warm-up, your primary aerobic session should not be done immediately before weight training.

Here is a sample home workout if you are a beginner at exercising. You will note that each day I am suggesting that you focus on a different part of the body: Day 1/Chest/Back/Trapezius (Monday); Day 2/Legs/Abs (Wednesday); Day 3/Arms (Friday). (You may also prefer to do these workouts on Tuesday, Thursday, and Saturday, with Wednesday, Friday, Sunday and Monday as your days off.

---

* Home refers to doing this workout on your own. You can do it at a local gym or health club, or in your home or apartment. Important note: This is general information only. Consult with your physician and work with a certified trainer, exercise physiologist or cardiac rehab nurse before beginning any exercise program or to customize these general workout programs.

Day 1 – Chest/Back/Trapezius (Monday)

Wide-grip push-ups against counter	3-4 sets of 12-15
Cable row with tubing	3-4 sets of 12-15
Cable forward press	3-4 sets of 12-15
Kneeling cable pulldown	3-4 sets of 12-15
Cable chest fly	3-4 sets of 12-15
One-arm bent-over dumbbell row	3-4 sets of 10-12
Dumbbell shrug	3-4 sets of 12-15

Stretching

Hold each stretch listed below at a point of a mild discomfort for 10-30 seconds. Repeat two to three times.

Chest stretch
Biceps stretch
Back stretch
Hanging back stretch
Alternate back stretch
Trapezius stretch
Neck stretch

Day 2 – Legs/Abs (Wednesday)

Wall squats on Swiss ball	3-4 sets of 12-15
Standing cable leg extension	3-4 sets of 12-15 each
Standing cable leg curl	3-4 sets of 12-15 each
Standing cable side hip extension	3-4 sets of 12-15 each
Standing calf raise on step	3-4 sets of 15
Cheat crunches on Swiss ball	3-4 sets of 15

Stretching
Quadriceps stretch
Hamstring/low back stretch
Feet-apart seated forward bend
Inner thigh stretch
Seated hip stretch
Calf stretch
Standing calf stretch

Oblique stretch

Day 3 – Arms (Friday)

External rotation with cables	3-4 sets of 12-15
Dumbbell standing front lateral raise	3-4 sets of 10-12
Dumbbell standing side lateral raise	3-4 sets of 10-12
Close-grip pushup against counter	3-4 sets of 12-15
One-arm dumbbell overhead triceps extension	3-4 sets of 10-12
Dumbbell biceps curl	3-4 sets of 10-12
Dumbbell hammer curl	3-4 sets of 10-12

Stretching
Shoulder stretch
Triceps stretch
Biceps stretch
Quadriceps stretch
Hamstring/low back stretch

Intermediate Home Workout

Aerobics can be performed three to seven days per week for 30 to 60 minutes. As noted above, if aerobics are done on the same day as resistance training, either perform the aerobics immediately after weight training or pick another time of day to do it. With the exception of five to 10 minutes of aerobics as a warm-up, your primary aerobic session should not be done immediately before weight training.

Day 1 – Chest/Back/Trapezius (Monday)

Dumbbell chest press on Swiss ball	3-4 sets of 8-10
Reverse-grip cable pulldown	3-4 sets of 12-15
Dumbbell fly on Swiss ball	3-4 sets of 10-12
Bent-over dumbbell row	3-4 sets of 8-10
Kneeling cable pullover	3-4 sets of 12-15
Dumbbell upright row	3-4 sets of 8-10
Swiss ball back extension	3-4 sets of 12-15

Stretching
Hold each stretch at a point of a mild discomfort for 10-30 seconds. Repeat 2-3 times.

Chest stretch
Biceps stretch
Back stretch
Hanging back stretch
Alternate back stretch
Trapezius stretch
Neck stretch

Day 2 – Legs/Abs (Wednesday)

Dumbbell squat	3-4 sets of 10-12
Dumbbell split squat	3-4 sets of 10-12
Stiff-legged deadlift	3-4 sets of 10-12
Cable hip adduction	3-4 sets of 12-15
Cable hip abduction	3-4 sets of 12-15
Single calf raise on step	3-4 sets of 10-12
Abdominal crunch on Swiss ball	3-4 sets of 12-15
V-ups	3-4 sets of 12-15

Stretching
Quadriceps stretch
Hamstring/low back stretch
Feet-apart seated forward bend
Inner thigh stretch
Seated hip stretch
Calf stretch
Standing calf stretch
Oblique stretch

Day 3 – Arms (Friday)

External rotation with cables	3-4 sets of 12-15
Dumbbell press on Swiss ball	3-4 sets of 8-10
One-arm dumbbell side lateral raise	3-4 sets of 10-12
One-arm dumbbell triceps kickback	3-4 sets of 10-12
Reverse-grip triceps extension	3-4 sets of 10-12

| Seated one-arm dumbbell concentration curl | 3-4 sets of 10-12 |
| Reverse-grip dumbbell curl | 3-4 sets of 8-10 |

Stretching
Shoulder stretch
Triceps stretch
Biceps stretch
Quadriceps stretch
Hamstring/low back stretch

Advanced Home Workout

As noted, aerobics can be performed three to seven days per week for 30 to 60 minutes. If aerobics are done on the same day as resistance training, either perform aerobics immediately after weight training or pick another time of day to do it. With the exception of five to 10 minutes of aerobics as a warm-up, your primary aerobic session should not be done immediately before weight training.

Day 1 – Chest/Back/Trapezius (Monday)

Dumbbell chest press on Swiss ball	3-4 sets of 6-10
Dumbbell chest fly on Swiss ball	3-4 sets of 8-10
Pushup	3-4 sets of max
Dumbbell deadlift	3-4 sets of 6-8
Bent-over dumbbell row	3-4 sets of 6-8
Kneeling cable pulldown	3-4 sets of 10-12
One-arm dumbbell row	3-4 sets of 6-8

Stretching
Hold each stretch at a point of a mild discomfort for 10-30 seconds. Repeat 2-3 times.

Chest stretch
Biceps stretch
Back stretch
Hanging back stretch
Alternate back stretch
Trapezius stretch
Neck stretch

Day 2 – Legs/Abs (Wednesday)

Dumbbell squat	3-4 sets of 6-8
Dumbbell walking lunge	3-4 sets of at least 10 each leg
Lying leg curl on Swiss ball	3-4 sets of 8-12
Single-leg stiff-legged deadlift	3-4 sets of 8-12
Sissy squat	3-4 sets of 12-15
Standing calf raise on step	1 set of 10-15 up each step
Weighted abdominal crunch on Swiss ball	3-4 sets of 12-15
Lying leg raise on Swiss ball	3-4 sets of max

Stretching
Quadriceps stretch
Hamstring/low back stretch
Feet-apart seated forward bend
Inner thigh stretch
Seated hip stretch
Calf stretch
Standing calf stretch
Oblique stretch

Day 3 – Arms (Friday)

Arnold press on Swiss ball	3-4 sets of 6-10
Bent-over rear dumbbell lateral raise	3-4 sets of 10-12
Standing dumbbell side lateral raise	3-4 sets of 8-10
Close-grip pushup	3-4 sets of max
Lying triceps extension on Swiss ball	3-4 sets of 8-10
1-arm dumbbell curl on Swiss ball	3-4 sets of 8-10
Standing alternate dumbbell curl	3-4 sets of 6-8

Stretching
Shoulder stretch
Triceps stretch
Biceps stretch
Quadriceps stretch
Hamstring/low back stretch

Chapter 10

*Exercise for Those with Heart Conditions
and Other Special Populations*

Up to this point, we've covered exercise guidelines with aerobic, anaerobic, and stretching routines to provide exceptional results. The target population was healthy individuals, as well as those with heart disease. In reality, few of us meet these categories. Many of us suffer from various diseases and/or disabilities, some of which go far beyond heart disease. Another population that needs addressing is those who have very recently suffered a heart attack and had a recent intervention. This chapter will provide adjustments to the workout routines, to meet the needs of those with one or more of these common ailments.

Exercise Considerations for Heart-Related Conditions

<u>Heart Attack</u>

For those who had recently suffered a heart attack, an intervention such as an angioplasty with or without a stent may have been done. Bypass surgery may have been performed, or a third possibility is that no intervention was performed and the cardiologist merely prescribed a medically-managed program which focuses on diet, medications and exercise to manage and, it is hoped, reverse heart disease.

Patients who have had an angioplasty with or without stents are usually instructed to wait one week before initiating or resuming an exercise program. They are instructed to watch their operation site for post-operative bleeding. This is usually the wrist or groin, depending on whether the radial or femoral artery was accessed. Additionally, patients are instructed to minimize stair climbing or lifting greater than 10 pounds for the first week after their procedure.

For those who recently had bypass surgery, they are usually instructed to avoid lifting objects heavier than five pounds for the first four weeks of their surgery. For the next four weeks, they can increase their intensity to a maximum of 10 pounds.

For the next four weeks, they have a 20-pound weight restriction. After 12 weeks post-op, they are free to lift whatever they can handle. It is at this point where they can have confidence that they will do no harm to their sternum from the incision. These patients usually begin an exercise program three to four weeks after hospital discharge, at the earliest. This is dependent upon how quickly they recovered after the procedure.

In my experience, I have found that people who are generally physically fit before the surgery tend to recover fastest.

Aerobic exercise is safe to perform at this time, but upper-extremity aerobics such as a rowing machine should be avoided for the full 12 weeks post-op, due to the amount of stress the chest area would be exposed to. Light resistance training can safely be performed, but should not isolate and emphasize the chest until ample healing time has passed.

For those who have recently suffered a heart attack and no intervention was done, it is usually safe to begin or resume exercise once medically stable after discharge from the hospital. These individuals would have no aerobic or weight restrictions that weren't already present before their heart attack.

The idea when starting or resuming any exercise program is to start slowly and progress at a steady pace. Rome was not built in a day and neither were your muscles.

During the cold, winter months in New England, I am frequently asked by my heart patients whether or not they can shovel snow. After all, it is a type of physical activity and I am constantly preaching about its importance. The fact of the matter is snow shoveling is not advised nor recommended for those with heart disease. Not only is the act of shoveling physically exerting by itself, breathing in the cold air adds another stress to your heart.

When we breathe in cold air, the blood vessels in our heart constrict, limiting the amount of oxygen-rich blood flow available. Couple that with the physical toll required and you significantly increase the likelihood of a future cardiac event. It's simply more stress on your heart than necessary. If the snow accumulation is only an inch or so and you feel you absolutely must go out and sweep or shovel the area, be sure to wear a scarf covering your nose and mouth to warm the cold air entering your lungs. But make no mistake, however, that this is ill-advised.

Stroke

A stroke, otherwise known as a cerebral vascular accident (CVA), is the result of insufficient blood flow to the brain. There are three different types of strokes. You can have a hemorrhagic stroke, often due to an aneurysm. You can have an ischemic stroke, where there is a lack of oxygen-rich blood flow to an area of the brain. You could also have a stroke due to a blood clot. With the lack of oxygen-rich blood to a part of the brain, cell death soon follows, with impairment in functioning of the central nervous system. It is basically a heart attack that occurs in the brain. It is commonly referred to as a "brain attack."

Several risk factors exist for developing a stroke: systolic and diastolic hypertension, diabetes mellitus, cigarette smoking, alcoholism and coronary artery disease. Other risk factors for heart disease may put one at risk for stroke as well. These risk factors include obesity and high cholesterol.[1]

The extent of neurological impairment from a stroke depends on the size of the blockage and location in the brain. You could have an impairment of the upper and/or lower extremities in terms of movement and/or sensation. You could have visual field defects, mental confusion, impaired speech, and/or impaired learning and performance of voluntary movements.

You don't have to be a rocket scientist to see how exercise can be a challenge for a stroke victim. You could have difficulty with movement due to weakness or developing spasticity of the extremities. Lacking adequate trunk balance may significantly limit options for exercise. Mental confusion may interfere with the ability to follow directions during exercise. Due to the advanced age of many stroke victims, other ailments may exist, such as coronary artery disease, arthritis, orthopedic issues, etc.

The few aerobic training studies done on stroke victims have shown significant improvements in terms of aerobic capacity.[1] The very deconditioned state stroke victims exhibit leaves much room for improvement. Studies have shown that people using assistive devices displayed greater mobility and less dependence on them. In rare cases, assistive devices were no longer required!

The goals of exercise with stroke victims should be not only to increase fitness levels, but also to focus on reducing risk factors, such as hypertension. Controlling blood pressure should be one of the major priorities for a stroke victim. Aerobic exercise kept at 40-70% of age-predicted maximum heart rate appears to be best for reducing hypertension. For those on heart-rate-reducing medications such as beta blockers, keeping an RPE between "3" and "4" should be adequate. Three days per week for 20-60 minutes per session should be sufficient.

The mode of exercise is dependent upon the individual's ability and whatever limitations are present. For example, someone with left arm and leg weakness may do well on an Airdyne˙ bike, where the right side can handle more of the load. The left side can go for the ride and may eventually show signs of improvement. If balance is an issue, the treadmill is probably not the best option. An arm bike or leg bike may work well. For those wheelchair bound, an arm bike is beneficial.

Similar to aerobic exercise, no exercise prescription for resistance training is set in stone for all stroke victims. Stroke victims can do only what is within their capabilities. Weight machines may be a safer option than free weights. Three sets of 8-12 repetitions on two days per week would be adequate.

Adding stretching to the aerobic and resistance training components would be wise. This can be performed both before and after the workouts. Balancing and coordination exercises can be beneficial, such as standing on one leg, quickly going from sitting to standing for multiple repetitions, and using a Swiss ball.

Exercise for Other Special Conditions

<u>Obesity</u>

Physical activity may be one of the most important factors in maintaining weight loss. This may be the result of increased caloric expenditure through exercise, or the positive behavior change exercise brings about, influencing decreased consumption of calories. I tend to think it's a combination of the two. The goal with exercise for the obese population is to reduce fat weight and preserve lean body weight (muscle).

For aerobic exercise, walking and/or non-weight-bearing exercise is best. These exercises should focus on working the major muscles of the lower body, and perhaps upper body as well. Examples would be the Airdyne˙ bike, NuStep˙, cross-trainer and treadmill.

Sessions should be daily or at least five days per week. They should last between 40 and 60 minutes. An intensity of 50-70% of maximum heart rate should be sufficient. Here, your main focus should be increasing duration before increasing intensity. It is fine to split up the session into two shorter ones of 20-30 minutes, if necessary.

A good way to progress is to start out at 20-30 minutes twice a day, at a low-moderate intensity of 50% of maximum heart rate, or about a "3" on the RPE scale.

Then, every two to three weeks, try increasing the duration by five minutes. Once you've gotten to 40 minutes, drop it down to one session per day and work your way towards 60 minutes daily.

It is important to note that excess body weight may exacerbate existing joint conditions. Therefore, it is especially wise to stick with low-impact or non-weight-bearing exercises and progress gradually in intensity and duration. Don't forget to include an adequate warm-up and cool-down, as well as stretching.

Another consideration is thermoregulation. Those with obesity are at an increased risk of heat intolerance.[1] To minimize this risk, exercise in a neutral environment, pick cool times of day to exercise, drink plenty of water, and wear loose-fitting clothing.

Resistance training is beneficial as an adjunct to aerobic training when trying to maintain or gain lean body mass. The idea here is to keep as much muscle mass as possible, to ensure that the weight you are losing is primarily fat. Two to four days per week of resistance training is adequate, following the same basic guidelines outlined for the general population.

Diabetes

An exercise program can provide those with diabetes a number of benefits. It can help lower blood glucose; improve insulin sensitivity, which will lower insulin requirements; reduce body fat, which further increases insulin sensitivity, in addition to providing cardiovascular benefits and stress reduction. Moreover, exercise can prevent type II diabetes in those at risk.[1]

The effect of diabetes on a single session of exercise depends on a number of factors, including blood glucose level before exercise; type of previous food intake, timing and amount eaten; type of exercise, duration, and intensity; type of glucose-lowering medication taken, and timing of medication. Another factor to consider is that if the body is under any additional stress, such as an illness, blood glucose levels may be affected. Appropriate care must be taken for adequate glucose management.

The exercise prescription for those with diabetes is similar to those without. However, there are some things worth taking into consideration. First of all, one hour of exercise requires an additional 15 grams of carbohydrates either before or immediately after. If exercise is of longer duration and higher intensity, an additional 15-30 grams of carbohydrate every hour may be necessary.[1] You will need to keep a source of fast-acting carbohydrate available during exercise. It is important to consume adequate fluids before, during and after exercise. Carrying a medical identification bracelet is a good idea as well. Practicing good foot care and wearing proper shoes and cotton socks is essential.

There are certain circumstances where exercise should be avoided. For example, if blood glucose is greater than 250 mg/dL and urinary ketones are present, exercise should be avoided until glucose is lowered.[1] The reason is that exercise under these circumstances may actually raise glucose further, instead of lowering it. The body is not able to burn sugar as energy, which could lead to more serious health problems. Another time to avoid exercise is when experiencing an illness or infection, which may further complicate glucose levels and insulin requirements. If blood glucose is 80-100 mg/dL, carbohydrates should be eaten with enough time for glucose to increase before exercise is initiated. The reason is a high risk of hypoglycemia. One other contraindication to exercise is an active retinal hemorrhage or recent therapy for retinopathy, which presents high risk of complications if exercising.

Exercise itself will ultimately be similar to those without diabetes. A 60-85% maximum heart rate is a good target for aerobics, but even 50% is fine. An RPE in the "3-5" range is also adequate. Thirty to 60 minutes per session is an appropriate target duration. Weight training two to four times per week would be wise. Maintain a stretching program at least three days per week. Use caution if exercising late in the evening, for the potential of hypoglycemia while sleeping. Plan for this with adequate carbohydrate consumption.

Arthritis

The two most common forms of arthritis are osteoarthritis (degenerative joint disease) and rheumatoid arthritis (an inflammatory disease affecting multiple joints and systems). Degenerative joint disease is localized to the affected joint or joints. Regardless of which type of arthritis is present, several consequences tend to result: people with arthritis tend to be less fit and less active than their unaffected peers; joint range of motion may be restricted due to pain, swelling, stiffness and bony changes. Those deconditioned, and those whose joints are poorly supported, are at increased risk of injury from high-impact or poorly controlled movements.

The greatest benefit exercise has to offer those with arthritis tends to be reducing the effects of inactivity. Problems common to both types of arthritis include loss of flexibility, muscle atrophy (shrinkage), weakness, osteoporosis, depression, fatigue and pain. These tend to be reduced with a low to moderate, gradually progressed exercise regime. It should be noted that, although it has beneficial effects for arthritics, exercise has not been shown to prevent or cure arthritis of any kind.[1]

There are several things those with arthritis need to consider with exercise. They should select low-impact exercises. Aerobic activities such as stair climbing, jogging and running are higher-impact exercises, and should be avoided, especially in those with hip or knee involvement with arthritis. Muscles need to be conditioned prior to more vigorous activity. A proper warm-up is essential, consisting of at least five minutes before more vigorous activity is implemented. Flexibility exercises are an important component that should be performed daily. Be careful to avoid overstretching, especially in unstable joints. Reduce the load on joints by selecting low-impact aerobic activities such as biking, rowing and swimming. Selecting a good pair of sneakers and insoles for maximum shock absorption during weight-bearing activities would be wise.

An exercise prescription for someone with arthritis would be doing low-impact aerobics three to five times per week, getting the target heart rate to 60-80% of age-predicted maximum, or an RPE of "3-5." Initially, use low intensity and duration. It may be as little as five minutes, building to 30 minutes per session. If necessary, accumulate the exercise in multiple bouts throughout the day. Using a *modified* interval training, consisting of brisk/rest exercise sessions, may be helpful as well. You can also try alternating pieces of aerobic equipment. For example, you can use the bike for 15 minutes, followed by the treadmill for another 15 minutes.

For strength training, avoid very heavy weights and high repetitions. Try keeping the repetitions to no greater than 12. Two to three days of resistance training is plenty. A good circuit training session, using a combination of free weights, machines and resistance bands, is appropriate.

Osteoporosis

After about 35 years of age, the activity of bone-forming cells begins to decline, leading to some minor loss of bone mass each year. Osteopenia is a condition of lowered bone mass. When osteopenia becomes severe enough that fractures occur due to a minimal amount of trauma, osteoporosis results. An example of this minimal trauma would be a broken hip related to a simple fall.

Evidence suggests regular exercise can slow or halt the age-related osteopenia and could delay the time point at which osteopenia progresses to osteoporosis.[1] There is no evidence that osteoporosis should alter the skeletal muscle and cardiovascular benefits of chronic exercise. Therefore, the recommended exercise program for those with osteoporosis is similar to the general exercise program for those with heart disease, with a few alterations.

Aerobics are recommended to be done three to five days per week, working at a target heart rate of 40-70% of age-predicted maximum heart rate, or "3-4" on RPE scale. Twenty to 30 minutes per session is adequate. Several modes of exercise (walking, biking, swimming) are acceptable, as long as forward flexion (bent over exercises) is minimized, because of the high risk of vertebral fractures in this population. If you're limited in your ability to perform weight-bearing activities due to multiple vertebral fractures, severe osteoporosis or back pain, select alternative exercises such as walking in the water, water aerobics, swimming and chair exercises.

Weight training should be incorporated two days per week; two to three sets of eight repetitions should be sufficient. You want to pick a weight appropriate for eight repetitions. Up to 40 minutes per workout is recommended for weight training. Keep in mind that those with vertebral fractures are likely to have decreased strength of the back extensor muscles. As a result, it is wise to start with low-intensity workouts, and progress slowly.

Stretching is important and should be done five to seven days per week. The goal is to increase and/or maintain range of motion, especially in the chest muscles. This will further reduce the likelihood of vertebral fractures.[1]

Keep in mind that it may take nine to 12 months of exercise before a change in the conservation of bone mass or lack thereof can be assessed. Try to be patient, and focus on perfect weight training form. Increase resistance as tolerated. Keep the exercise area free from clutter, to further reduce the risk of injury related to falls.

Chronic Pulmonary Disease

Chronic pulmonary disease can be divided up into two major categories: obstructive and restrictive pulmonary disease. In obstructive pulmonary disease, the airways tend to become smaller during expiration, due to an airflow obstruction. As a result, lung volume decreases. Chronic bronchitis and asthma are examples of this. Restrictive pulmonary disease is a type of lung disease in which there is reduced lung compliance. Examples of this are pulmonary fibrosis and emphysema. Although other pulmonary disorders exist, these obstructive and restrictive disorders tend to be more common, and will be our focus here.

With chronic pulmonary disease, cardiovascular deconditioning is an inevitable consequence of reduced physical activity. Muscular fatigue due to lactic acid buildup results in low exercise work rate. Peripheral muscles become deconditioned as well. Muscle wasting and weakness result, due to physical inactivity and malnutrition. Long-term glucocorticoid use (i.e. Prednisone), commonly prescribed for COPD and pulmonary fibrosis, also contribute to muscle wasting. Anxiety and depression tend to be a factor related to chronic pulmonary disease, due to the frightening nature of the symptoms and the inability to pursue some normal activities of daily living.

Exercise in this population is crucial. It will provide cardiovascular reconditioning; improve strength, flexibility and body composition; and provide a decreased feeling of breathlessness.[1] Although exercise can help the individual reach a higher level of physical activity, it won't take long for physical deconditioning to result, due to a relapse of low activity. Therefore, it is crucial to maintain a high level of physical activity on most, if not all, days of the week.

Aerobic exercise should be done three to seven days per week, for at least 30 minutes per session. Shorter bouts may be used, as long as they add up to 30 minutes in a day. Focus on exercises that use the large muscles of your body (i.e. walking, cycling, swimming). Your rate of perceived exertion should be "3-4" on the RPE scale. Emphasis should be on increasing the duration of aerobic exercise before addressing intensity.

Resistance training should be done two to three days per week. The focus should be on increasing the maximal number of repetitions, as opposed to maximal weight. Two to three sets of 10-15 repetitions per exercise should be sufficient.

Stretching should be done at least three times per week. The focus should be on large muscle groups, such as legs and lower back. Stretch the specific muscle groups exercised that day.

RPE and the degree of shortness of breath should be the methods used to monitor intensity. Heart rate will not be the best indicator, since most people with chronic pulmonary disease are not able to achieve a *training* exercise heart rate. It would be wise to avoid extremes in temperature and humidity. People with chronic pulmonary disease tend to respond to exercise best in mid- to late morning.

Respiratory symptoms seem to be worst first thing in the early morning. If supplemental oxygen is used, it should be adjusted to maintain an oxygen saturation of >90%. Pursed lip breathing is a technique that can help slow the respiratory rate. To accomplish this, narrow the space between your lips as you exhale. An improvement should be seen in breathing efficiency.

Cancer

Cancer is a disease in which there is abnormal cell growth, with the potential for these cells to spread to other anatomical sites. It is not a single disease. Instead, it is a collection of hundreds of diseases that share the distinction of abnormal cell growth.

Treatment for cancer involves surgery, chemotherapy and/or radiation. A person is considered cancer-free if he or she is in remission. Remission is not always possible, since the potential exists for a few cancer cells to escape being eradicated, and eventually grow back. Patients in remission as well as those undergoing treatment can benefit from regular exercise training.

For those in remission, the goal of exercise should be to return to their previous physical and psychological level of functioning. For those currently receiving chemotherapy or radiation, the goal of exercise should be to maintain strength, endurance, and their current level of functioning. These people are usually easily fatigued and worn out from their cancer treatments. Some side effects of chemotherapy and radiation can be permanent. They have the potential for causing permanent scar formation in joints, as well as in heart and lung tissue. Another possibility is drug-induced cardiomyopathy, which can cause a permanent decline in cardiovascular functioning. Surgery can cause pain, loss of flexibility, possibly amputation, as well as motor and sensory nerve damage.

Some major benefits that exercise can have in cancer survivors are increased skeletal muscle strength and endurance, as well as a boost in psychological status. The goal of exercise for cancer survivors is to return to a healthy, active lifestyle. For those in therapy, the focus should be on improving strength, endurance and psychological status. In some cases, slowing down or preventing muscle wasting is the main objective.

The exercise prescription for the cancer patient is (and *must be*) unique to the individual. No set guidelines exist, because people suffer from different types of cancer, are at different stages, require different treatments, etc. An exercise program should include an aerobic component, a strength-training, and a flexibility component. It is important to avoid training to exhaustion, especially in those undergoing therapy. My recommendation would be to try the basic exercise program I've outlined, and make adjustments as you feel necessary. Focus more on RPE as opposed to attempting to reach a target heart rate, with aerobic exercise. Listen to your body and give yourself sufficient rest periods when necessary.

Chapter 11

Pain: The Good, the Bad, and the 911

It would be naïve to think that you could go through life being free from illness and injury. Various illnesses or injuries tend to plague us all from time to time, often during the most inconvenient of times, whether it is a common cold or flu or even something more debilitating, like a broken arm or torn muscle. Believe it or not, some injuries are considered normal with exercise, and can actually be beneficial. When we exercise at a high intensity, we are actually damaging muscle cells. It is this process that enables the muscles to grow bigger and stronger. The purpose of this chapter is to identify different types of injuries that are possible with exercise, and determine the best action to take in order to promote the quickest and most efficient healing time. I will also differentiate *good pain* from *bad pain*.

What is "Normal" Exercise Soreness?

To determine what is abnormal, we must first have a clear understanding of what is normal when it comes to soreness. Muscle soreness is a type of pain present at specific muscles during the latter stages of an exercise bout, during the immediate recovery period, between 12 and 48 hours after a strenuous exercise bout, or at all of the above times.

There are two basic types of muscle soreness: *acute muscle soreness* and *delayed onset muscle soreness (DOMS)*.

Acute muscle soreness is the pain felt during and immediately after exercise; it can result from accumulation of the end products of exercise, such as lactic acid, and from tissue swelling caused by fluid shifting from blood plasma into the tissues. This is that *pumped up* feeling you get after a heavy endurance or strength-training session. This is actually a *normal* sensation that usually disappears anywhere from within a few minutes to several hours after exercise.

How can you effectively deal with this normal situation? I remember trying to play basketball within a couple of hours after training my chest and arms. The ball felt like a boulder every time I attempted a shot. Needless to say, I learned rather quickly to avoid activities combining physical activity with hand-eye coordination so soon after lifting.

Muscle soreness felt a day or two after a heavy bout of exercise is known as delayed onset muscle soreness (DOMS). Although several theories exist as to why DOMS occurs, more research is needed before the exact reason can be determined. It appears to mainly result from eccentric action and is associated with actual muscle damage.[1] Eccentric movements are those in which the muscle is stretched or lengthened when resistance is applied. An example would be the lowering phase of a biceps curl. The presence of muscle enzymes in blood after intense exercise supports the notion that some structural damage may occur in the muscle membranes. Experts generally agree that this damage is partly responsible for the localized muscle pain, tenderness and swelling connected with DOMS. Some evidence suggests that the process of muscle damage is an important step in muscle hypertrophy.

With DOMS comes a pain that can last from a few days to as much as a couple of weeks, gradually decreasing in intensity. The soreness also brings a decrease in the force-generating capacity of the affected muscle. As a result, you tend to have muscle weakness, which gradually resolves over a period of days to weeks. I often experience DOMS once I resume exercise after a rest period of a few weeks or greater. Just the act of sitting in a chair can be quite challenging. Every so often, one of my patients will complain of how sore their arms or legs are after their workouts with me. Neither the complaining nor the soreness last too long before the patient is pleasantly surprised at the new strength they were able to muster.

What is important to recognize is that DOMS is quite normal. It can be painful at the specific muscles that were trained, but it can be referred to as *good pain*. Stretching immediately after exercise may reduce the intensity of the discomfort, but rest is what ultimately relieves it. This is not to say you should avoid activity completely. You should just rest those specific muscles until the soreness resolves itself, so you have the necessary strength returned to those muscles.

One method of reducing DOMS is to train at a low intensity for a couple of weeks, and gradually increase workout intensity. Another approach is to train intensely early on, get the DOMS and with subsequent training bouts, less and less muscle soreness would result. Because of the potential connection between DOMS and muscle hypertrophy, DOMS may be necessary to maximize the training response; especially if increasing muscle size is an objective.

Recognizing and coping with "bad pain"

Now that we've covered the *good pain*, it's time to investigate what makes up *bad pain*. Injuries can be so slight and so common that we tend to ignore them. The phrase "walk it off" was a common saying on the court when I was a college tennis player. Other injuries, however, can be more serious and require medical attention. We will discuss some of the more common injuries and how to treat them.

<u>Strains and tears</u>
One type of injury common to the exerciser is a strain. This could be a muscle strain, a strain in the tendons, or where tendon connects to bone. It is often caused by overworking these structures or by a single violent episode, such as a sudden stretching force applied to a muscle that is vigorously contracting. If that force is greater than what the muscle or tendon can handle, a tear may result. This can be a partial tear or a complete tear. A partial tear is usually mild.

A partial tear is sometimes referred to as a pulled muscle. The result would be pain and discomfort with movement. Muscle spasms may also occur. When partial tears are more severe, symptoms are increased with swelling and limited movement, in addition to increased pain.

The initial treatment for partial tears is rest, ice, compression, elevation and stabilization. Think of the acronym "RICES." You want to rest the injured area because trying to work through the injury can only make things worse, increasing the chances of turning that partial tear into a complete tear. Ice will be beneficial not only to help numb the initial pain, but also to cause vasoconstriction of the blood vessels, which limits blood flow to the area, reducing hemorrhaging and inflammation.

Compression is also beneficial for similar reasons. Elevating the extremity is important to help blood flow out of the injured area. Stabilization is used to limit movement, thus preventing further injury. Simply put, you want the area immobilized for a few days.

Within a few days, you should experience more freedom of movement with less pain. These partial tears tend to require four to eight weeks for full recovery. You may feel you'd be able to exercise the injured area after about two weeks. This is usually fine, as long as the workout is kept light with slow progression, week by week. The main objective here is to allow complete recovery and prevent further injury.

In severe muscle and tendon injuries with a complete tear, surgical repair is usually necessary. Even in these severe cases, initial treatment will be similar to a partial tear, using RICES. When in doubt whether it's a partial or complete tear, it may be wise to seek medical attention. If it's fairly obvious that it's a partial tear (i.e. no physical deformity observed, no pain at rest), using RICES should be sufficient.

Muscle spasms and cramps tend to be another sign of a strain. A spasm or cramp is nothing more than a sudden, violent, involuntary muscle contraction, which can be quite painful. You can think of it as a protective mechanism of the body against further motion until there has been sufficient recovery time. I tend to get abdominal spasms when training my abdominals, which can be pretty painful. It would often feel like knives were being stabbed into my midsection with only the slightest shifts in position. They can be very short and mild, or may last for several days with more pain. The spasms of short duration are usually cramping related to overuse and fatigue. Rest and protecting the area against further injury are usually all that is required. My abdominal spasms forced me to take about four weeks off from abdominal work and slowly reintroduced the abdominal exercises back in my regime with great success. I would start off by doing one set of one exercise twice a week and make an increase every week until I had reached three sets of two abdominal exercises.

In eleven years of being involved with cardiac rehab, I've had only one incident in which a client experienced a muscle strain. He was in his early 70s and was helping another participant rack his 30-pound dumbbells. This gentleman was so strong for his age, these heavy dumbbells were nothing unreasonable for him to use. When handed the 30-pound dumbbell, he was in an awkward position and immediately felt a pop. He suffered a partial tear (strain) of his right biceps. The injury looked pretty bad the next day, due to his blood-thinning medication, Plavix, which showed dark bruising covering the majority of his upper arm. Despite how bad it looked, it wasn't too painful as long as he didn't stress it by lifting weights. He was compliant by resting and icing the injured extremity. Within two months, he was back to working his biceps with no problems or limitations.

Tendonitis

Tendonitis is another overuse injury common to the exerciser. This is an inflammation of the synovium, which lines a tendon sheath and surrounds the tendon. Pain is usually present just with movement, but depending on the location, it could also occur at rest. In the early stages of tendonitis, the treatment is similar to that for a muscle strain, where rest and protection against further injury are important. As the saying goes, "if it hurts, don't do it."

With minor episodes of tendonitis, pain usually resolves within a couple of weeks. In advanced stages, complications tend to be more serious and may require surgery. Corticosteroids are sometimes used (e.g. cortisone injection) to minimize the pain by reducing the inflammation process. Unfortunately, the success rate may be as little as 30% of those that get it experiencing relief.[2]

Several studies have shown cortisone injections to be associated with short-term benefits, but within six to 18 months, symptoms tend to worsen in the majority of sufferers.[3,4]

I've worked with patients who have had cortisone injections for episodes of tendonitis, as well as for arthritis. Some have experienced success, while others either had no success or had temporary relief lasting only days or weeks.

Every so often, I'll work with a patient in cardiac rehab who is dealing with tendonitis. The most common location I've seen it is in the inner forearm, usually related to heavy dumbbell bicep curls. They may have tried to progress too much too fast. When it flares up, I instruct patients to stop the exercise until the pain completely goes away (generally two to four weeks). I find alternative exercises to work the muscle without causing additional discomfort to the tendons. I remind the patient that if it hurts, don't do it!

I am no stranger to tendonitis, either. I had a bout of quadriceps tendonitis, which gave me intense pain at both knee caps. I was fine at rest, but to squat down with my own bodyweight gave me such excruciating pain that I would need to hold onto a stable object to get myself back up. Although I was avoiding squats and lunges in my leg workouts, I found I could do fewer and fewer exercises without experiencing the knee pain as weeks and months progressed. Ice, stretching and rest did not seem to help.

What ultimately did help was a one-hour deep-tissue massage, focusing specifically on the quadriceps, hamstrings and calves. Immediately after the session, I was miraculously able to squat again. Whether the massage loosened tight muscles or broke up scar tissue, which enhanced blood flow to the area, the important thing is that I found a solution to the problem. To prevent a relapse, I slowly progressed from squatting light to squatting heavy.

All was well with the tendons until about two years later when the pain returned shortly after a strenuous leg workout; perhaps the weight was too heavy or my form was less than perfect. Either way, I figured another deep-tissue massage would fix this in a hurry. To my surprise, it offered no relief! Desperate for a remedy, I saw an orthopedic surgeon, who gave me options: I could take a cortisone injection which could relieve the pain, but could also weaken the joint and increase susceptibility to a complete tear in the future. The other option was platelet-rich plasma therapy (PRPT).

PRPT is an injection of the patient's own blood into the injured area in order to "jump start" the body's instincts to repair muscle, bone and other tissue. The procedure starts off with a small sample of blood taken from the patient. This blood goes through a machine that spins really fast to separate blood components and isolate the platelets. About one to two teaspoons of this platelet-enriched plasma is injected into the injured area. The theory is that, with all the growth factors and proteins involved in the healing process present in the injured area in such high concentrations, healing time will be drastically reduced. This could be extremely therapeutic in areas with poor blood supply, such as tendons and ligaments.

Other benefits of PRPT are that, since it uses the patient's own blood, there is less chance of infection than a surgical incision, it leaves no scar, and there is quicker recovery time compared to surgery. It also shouldn't weaken the joint as cortisone injections could. Several professional athletes have already experienced great success with PRPT for tendon and ligament issues, although more studies are needed to prove its effectiveness in this area.[5]

Desperate for pain relief, I opted to give PRPT a try. Although the injections were quite painful in both knees, after eight days of "resting the knees," pain was miraculously gone! I could now squat and lunge with my own body weight without pain! After two weeks of rest, I resumed aerobics on a recumbent bike. After two months of rest from leg training, I resumed my leg workouts, with no problems ever since.

Although various methods of treatment may help, the most important method for successful recovery from tendonitis is rest. Again: If it hurts, don't do it. Wait until the pain is relieved before reintroducing the exercise and slowly progress with weight. You're only as strong as your weakest link. The muscle tends to adapt quicker than the tendon. Respect your body and it will be good to you in return.

Sprain

Another injury an exerciser may face is a sprain. A sprain is an injury to a ligament, usually from overstress, resulting in damage to the substance of the ligament or attachment site. It's commonly caused by a violent external force that causes the joint to move in an awkward direction, which stresses the ligament beyond its ability to withstand tearing. Think of it like this: strains involve muscles and tendons, whereas sprains generally deal with ligaments. Ligaments are tough fibrous bands which connect two bones.

Treatment for sprains is not very different than treatment for strains. Course of treatment depends on the severity of the sprain. Initial action would be to rest the area and stabilize it. You may need to splint the area and/or apply a compression dressing. Ice would be beneficial, especially for the first 48 hours. This will promote vasoconstriction (narrowing of the blood vessels), which will limit inflammation. Elevating the injured extremity is also important to promote adequate blood return to the heart and further reduce inflammation.

Sprains are the type of injury you don't want to work through. Your best chance of complete recovery is to wait until you are pain-free before resuming those particular exercises. If it is a minor sprain with not a great deal of pain and inflammation, the RICES treatment should be sufficient.

For more severe sprains with more bleeding and swelling, more pain with joint motion and greater loss of joint function, seeing an orthopedist is best. This will ensure there are no broken bones or potential complete rupture of the ligament. X-rays would be needed to rule this out. The severity of the sprain would determine the length of recovery time. The key things to remember for a sprain as well as for a strain are to avoid working the injured area until pain-free, and remember the acronym RICES.

To clarify, sprains are not a common injury in the type of exercise promoted in this book. In over 18 years of training, I've suffered a total of two sprains. The first sprain was of my index finger while playing basketball. The second was a sprained knee while playing high school football. The reason I mention this type of injury is not so much because you'll be at risk with this type of exercise, but because you may experience sprains through other means, forcing you to adjust your workouts accordingly.

Sickness
There tends to be confusion and perhaps some guilt regarding when it's beneficial to train while sick and when it's best to skip the workout, especially once you have an exercise routine established and you are reluctant to "break" your schedule.

You first need to differentiate between different types of sickness. You can have your common head cold, which usually will show symptoms from the neck up. You may experience a sore throat, headache, stuffy nose and/or cough. Under these conditions, it's safe to exercise. You may actually feel a decrease in severity of symptoms after a workout. Whether there's a physiological reason for this or just a psychological benefit related to elevated endorphins remains unclear. What is important to note is that your body temperature should be less than or equal to 99.5 degrees F. With a temperature greater than 99.5, rest would be advised to prevent increasing the severity of the illness. If the cold affects any area from below the neck (i.e. chest, stomach), exercise is not recommended.[6] It would be wise to rest and try again another day. Based on this information, exercise should be avoided when suffering from the flu.

In my eighteen years of training, I can recall numerous occasions exercising when I was sick. Breathing would be so challenging, I'd feel as if two golf balls were wedged in my nostrils. More often than not, I'd actually experience fairly productive workouts under such circumstances. In fact, I'd often feel significantly better after working up a sweat, where I'd feel my breathing had improved. Although these improvements would rarely last long, I felt more energetic and productive after exercise, despite being sick.

The times I couldn't train were when experiencing flu-like symptoms. There were times where my body ached as if I were on the losing end of a fistfight. My ambitious nature had gotten the best of me at times, and I would think I could just "sweat away" the fever. This would often leave me feeling worse the following day, having less energy with possibly even a rise in body temperature. If gastrointestinal issues were involved, I'd end up spending more time in the bathroom than in the squat rack!

These days, I do a better job of listening to my body. If I'm dealing with a sniffle, cough and/or sore throat, I won't hesitate to train at my usual intensity. If my temperature is above 99.5, especially if associated with fatigue, body aches and pains, and possibly gastrointestinal symptoms, I'm taking the day off and resting appropriately. I may even extend this rest period to a week or more to ensure my immune system can properly handle such physical exertion.

The reason colds, in particular, should be of concern to those with heart disease is because of potential complications. Pneumonia is a complication in which it becomes increasingly difficult to take in oxygen efficiently. This forces the heart to work harder, pumping oxygen-rich blood throughout the body more forcefully.

It is important to be aware of certain cold medicines, especially for those suffering from heart disease, and to consider avoiding those containing decongestants such as "pseudoephedrine" or "phenylephrine." These ingredients will raise blood pressure, forcing the heart to work harder by constricting blood vessels, which reduces swelling in the nose and opens nasal passages. These ingredients also interfere with numerous prescription medications.

Non-steroidal anti-inflammatory drugs (NSAIDs) such as ibuprofen which are often used to relieve cold symptoms may also not be the best drugs of choice. Among other side effects, NSAIDs can cause fluid retention. In those suffering from congestive heart failure, this will only intensify the condition.

One apparently safe option for cold medicine is Coricidin HBP' but you still want to check out if it is okay to take this and exercise by consulting your physician if you have a heart condition. This is a decongestant-free over-the-counter cold medicine. It contains an antihistamine and cough suppressant.

Several forms of this cold medicine also contain acetaminophen (Tylenol), to act as a fever reducer. Once again, it would be wise to check with your doctor before starting this medicine, to ensure it won't interfere with other prescribed medications.

For those suffering from heart disease, it's best to prevent colds whenever possible. Good hygiene is key. Hand washing is the single most important thing you can do to help prevent the spread of respiratory infections such as colds. Regular exercise, eating a nutritious diet and limiting stress are all effective measures to ensure peak performance of your immune system.

Overtraining

A potential problem affecting exercisers is overtraining. Overtraining is an unexplained decline in performance, which can be connected to physiological and psychological causes. It tends to occur when exercise is too intense for too long, with insufficient recovery time. It is very difficult to recognize because the symptoms are unique to the individual and often very subtle. The first sign of overtraining is usually a decrease in performance. The exerciser may feel significantly weaker, with loss of muscular strength, stamina and/or coordination. Other symptoms that may be present are weight loss and decreased appetite, elevated heart rate and blood pressure, sleep disturbances, increased susceptibility to colds, and muscle tenderness. Psychological issues related to overtraining include fatigue and a loss of enthusiasm to train.

Although the exact cause of overtraining is not fully understood, most researchers agree that there is physical and/or emotional overload, which might trigger the condition. Because many of the symptoms of overtraining are vague and can have a number of other etiologies, it is very hard to detect. The exerciser generally doesn't experience any early warning signs.

The only way to overcome this condition is with days, and in some cases weeks, of reduced exercise or complete rest. Cycle your training with days of easier workouts, moderate and harder periods. A good rule is to follow one or two hard workouts with an equal number of easier training sessions.

My worst overtraining experience to date occurred three months after competing in a 2009 national bodybuilding competition. I failed to get the placing I felt I'd deserved. Eager to come back in even better shape next year, I quickly resumed my vigorous training. I was a man on a mission.

I took only two weeks off weight training before resuming my hectic workout schedule. The muscles were starving for a much longer rest, but my misguided exuberance led me to push my body further. As a result, I ended up tearing my left biceps and right hamstring muscles (muscle strains), in addition to the dreaded return of my troublesome quadriceps tendonitis. Not realizing it was torn, I continued training the biceps for another three weeks! I just remember feeling an uncomfortable tightness that seemed to intensify over several weeks. It wasn't until tearing my hamstring muscle that I finally accepted the fact that I had pushed my body well over its limit. Had this happened to a friend or client of mine, I could've spotted it in a heartbeat.

I allowed my exercise zeal and focus to supersede my better judgment and overall health. It took 10 weeks of inactivity before I could consider returning to training. Upon my return, I needed a good four weeks of light training before returning to the intensity I had become accustomed to.

It is essential to be aware of how you're feeling, both at rest and with exercise. Whether you are carrying groceries, walking the dog or exercising moderately-to-vigorously on a bike, you need to be aware of what's normal so you can take appropriate measures if you experience something abnormal. This following section will make you aware of abnormal signs and symptoms, the significance of each (e.g. cardiovascular, pulmonary or metabolic disease), and when to seek medical attention.

Angina

This is a specific pain, located in the chest, neck, arms, jaw, forearms, fingers and/or upper back area which may result from a lack of oxygen-rich blood flow to the heart. This is not a pain provoked by a specific body motion, nor is it aggravated by respiration. This is a burning, squeezing, heavy feeling. It can be brought on by exercise, stress, cold weather or excitement, or may occur after meals. This could represent a classic case of angina, where oxygen-rich blood is not adequately supplied to a certain area of the heart. If this has not been diagnosed, you need to take action. In addition to calling 911, if no contraindication (e.g. allergy) exists, chew a regular-strength 325 mg aspirin. This will help thin your blood to improve circulation. If you have been previously diagnosed with angina and take sublingual nitroglycerin as needed, take one tablet. If after five minutes chest pain remains, take another tablet and wait an additional five minutes. If pain remains, take one more tablet. Call 911 if pain remains after a total of three tablets have been taken.[7,8]

Shortness of Breath

Shortness of breath can occur at rest or with mild exertion. This is suggestive of cardiac or pulmonary disease. This is normal with healthy in-shape individuals exercising at a high intensity, or even untrained individuals exercising at a lower intensity. This becomes a problem if shortness of breath occurs at a lower intensity level, where you normally would not be short of breath. An example would be being short of breath while warming up on the treadmill. If you notice something like this, it would be wise to call your doctor.

Dizziness & Syncope

Dizziness is simply feeling lightheaded. At the very least, dizziness can occur in healthy people shortly after exercise, as a result of reduced venous blood return to the heart. This may be evident when finishing an aerobic workout on the treadmill: as soon as the belt stops, you feel like you're on a boat, rocking from side to side. This lightheadedness usually goes away after about 30 seconds, and generally is of little concern.

Another possible explanation for dizziness is too high a dosage in blood pressure medications, where blood pressure is too low. A long-term benefit of exercise is achieving a lower blood pressure. If you're currently taking a blood pressure medication, the dose may need to be adjusted. It's best to notify your physician of this.

Syncope is defined as loss of consciousness; simply, in other words, passing out. It's most commonly caused by reduced blood flow to the brain. Dizziness and particularly syncope during exercise may result from potentially life-threatening cardiac disorders. These symptoms should not be ignored. If you were to experience syncope, regardless of whether or not you are exercising, seek medical attention immediately. Get yourself checked out at a walk-in medical center or an emergency department. This is not the time to schedule an appointment with your cardiologist or general practitioner three or four weeks later.

Orthopnea & Paroxysmal Nocturnal Dyspnea

Orthopnea is defined as shortness of breath at rest in a lying position, and is relieved by sitting upright or standing. Paroxysmal nocturnal dyspnea is a sudden shortness of breath that usually occurs after a few hours of sleep and is relieved by sitting on the side of the bed or standing up. Both can be symptoms of a dysfunction of the left ventricle of the heart, which can be quite serious. This shortness of breath is different from that of one with chronic obstructive pulmonary disease (COPD) in that coughing and relieving secretions usually relieve the shortness of breath if it's a COPD issue.

Intermittent Claudication

Intermittent claudication is a pain that occurs in a muscle with reduced blood flow when exercising. The pain does not occur at rest, and is reproducible with a certain level of physical activity. It's commonly described as a cramp and usually resolves after a minute or two of rest. It frequently occurs in the legs, whether in calves or upper thighs. It can be diagnosed as peripheral vascular disease (PVD). People with diabetes are at increased risk of developing this. I've worked with a number of clients suffering with it, and in many cases, regular exercise has increased their ability to train longer and at a higher intensity. If this is a new pain for you, it would be wise to contact your physician for a proper diagnosis. In more severe cases, medical and surgical treatments are available.

Palpitations & Tachycardia

Palpitations can be defined as an unpleasant awareness of the forceful or rapid beating of the heart. Tachycardia can be defined as a heart rate greater than 100 bpm. You can have what's referred to as supraventricular tachycardia (SVT) which is an arrhythmia in which the normal pacemaker of the heart is replaced by other pacemakers in the atria, generating a heart rate >150 bpm (see figure 12 in chapter 3, "Heart-related Illnesses, Tests, and Treatments").

There are many other arrhythmias that can present themselves, such as atrial fibrillation and ventricular tachycardia. These can be quite serious and require immediate medical attention. One way to check to see if this *feeling* of palpitations is valid is to check your pulse. Place your index finger and middle finger over your radial artery (one inch below your thumb) or carotid artery (the side of your neck).

Count the pulsations as you look at the hands of a clock and count for one minute. If you notice that beats are greater than 100 bpm and/or an irregular beat pattern that is new for you, it would be wise to call your doctor or go to the emergency department, where a 12-lead EKG can be done.

Ankle Edema

Bilateral ankle edema (swelling in both ankles) can be most evident at night and is a characteristic sign of heart failure, due to insufficient venous blood flow in both legs. Edema is swelling, usually due to fluid retention. A classic sign that it could be heart failure would be shortness of breath and fatigue, along with the ankle edema.

If you have recently gained a significant amount of weight in a very short time (e.g. greater than five lbs. in two days), this may be cause for concern. A classic sign of ankle edema is the presence of sock marks on your legs.

Additionally, you can try pressing a finger against your ankle/shin area. If you notice an indentation, you are retaining fluid in your lower extremities.

If you have edema in only one limb, it's often the result of a clot in a blood vessel. You could also have generalized edema throughout your body, referred to as anasarca. This can occur in those with severe heart failure, or serious kidney or liver disease. Under these conditions, your physician should be notified.

In summary, the purpose of this chapter was not meant to scare you of the potential dangers of exercise. Granted, there are risks associated with all of the exercises described in this book. There are also risks associated with climbing up and down a flight of stairs. This chapter was meant to provide clarity and understanding as to what is normally experienced with exercise, as well as what is abnormal. The fact is exercise can help reduce many of the listed ailments, such as hypertension, obesity and diabetes, which can lead to more serious conditions like CHF, strokes, osteoporosis and heart attacks.

Most valuable of all is to be aware of how you're feeling. When your body tells you to do more, wisely listen to it. When your body tells you that you should slow down or stop, it's important to be attentive and follow your body's lead. Listen to your body; it's usually right.

Part 3

Additional Considerations

Chapter 12

Understanding Your Medications
and Their Implications For Your Exercise Routines

Few of us can get through life without being prescribed at least one medication to control various ailments we might be faced with, whether hypertension, high cholesterol, diabetes or arthritis. Although the majority of these medications have no effect on our exercise performance, there are certain medications that will. In some cases, exercise will alter the dosages of medications required. In this chapter, we will review some of the more common medications and important points to consider if you are taking a particular medication when you are exercising.

Anticoagulants

Anticoagulants are blood thinners. By interfering with the blood's natural clotting system, they help prevent clots from forming within blood vessels as well as slowly dissolving those that may have already formed.

Most anticoagulants are given via injection; either intravenously or subcutaneously. Heparin˙ and Lovenox˙ are two examples. If administered subcutaneously or within the fatty layer under your skin, the optimum injection site is in the belly, where we tend to store more subcutaneous fat. Warfarin (Coumadin˙) is an oral (pill) form of an anticoagulant. Anticoagulants are used to treat various blood clots, unstable angina or a heart attack, as well as to prevent strokes in patients with mechanical heart valves and patients with atrial fibrillation or blood clots in the heart chambers.[1]

The majority of patients taking anticoagulants are on Coumadin˙, since it is the most readily available oral form. It is a very potent anticoagulant which prevents harmful clots from forming or increasing in size. While the patient is on the drug, blood work needs to be done regularly, on average once every couple of weeks, to ensure clotting factors and clotting time are in an acceptable range.

There are many restrictions for those taking Coumadin˙. Foods high in vitamin K (broccoli, spinach, cabbage, Brussels sprouts, etc.) need to be limited. You don't have to refrain from eating them completely, but you must stay consistent with whatever amount you currently eat. Otherwise, your clotting factors will be inconsistent, which will make it impossible for your doctor to determine the proper dosage of Coumadin˙.

Be aware of other foods and food supplements if you are taking Coumadin˙. For example, many multivitamins contain Vitamin K. It would be wise to read the listing of ingredients and find a multivitamin that does not include Vitamin K.

Xarelto® and Pradaxa® are two newer alternatives to Coumadin® which do not require the same frequency of blood tests or Vitamin K restrictions. Blood work should be done prior to starting either of these medications, and at least once annually, to ensure excess stress has not been placed on your kidneys. It is important to note that with Xarelto® and Pradaxa®, there is no reversal agent, other than hemodialysis. This is in contrast to Coumadin®, where Vitamin K can reverse its blood-thinning effects.

Regardless of the anticoagulant taken, it is important to avoid hazardous activities, such as playing football or hockey, as well as any other dangerous work. Be careful to avoid activities with a high risk of bleeding injuries because once the bleeding starts, it can be difficult to stop. Be sure to report any signs of bleeding, such as under the skin, as well as in urine, stool, and gums. Speaking of gums, it is important to inform your dentist and other physicians if you are taking an anticoagulant. Use a soft-bristle toothbrush to avoid bleeding gums as well as an electric razor for shaving.

Unfortunately, neither Xarelto® nor Pradaxa® are effective for treatment of heart valve problems. But it is being used to minimize the risk of stroke associated with atrial fibrillation. For those with heart valve problems, Coumadin® remains the drug of choice.

Whether you are on Coumadin®, Xarelto®, or Pradaxa®, switching from one anticoagulant to another is a serious decision that should be made with your cardiologist. If you plan to have any type of surgical procedure, you will need approval from your cardiologist, as well as instructions on how to adjust your anticoagulant, in order to prevent excessive bleeding.

Antiplatelet Agents

Platelets are small cells in the bloodstream that promote clotting. Antiplatelet agents prevent platelets from doing their job. This provides a mild form of blood thinning. Antiplatelet agents are used to treat patients with unstable angina and heart attack, as well as stable heart patients. They prolong the survival of heart attack victims, reduce the risk of repeat strokes in those who've had a stroke or mini-stroke, and improve the outcome of angioplasties and stent placement.[1]

One of the most common antiplatelet agents is aspirin. Unless there are contraindications, such as an allergy or the use of a more potent blood thinner, heart patients are generally prescribed aspirin on a daily basis. A common dose is anywhere from 81 mg to 325 mg.

From an exercise standpoint, if you are taking a daily aspirin, you shouldn't have anything to be concerned with. However, another reason aspirin may be prescribed is for its anti-inflammatory properties, which are unique to aspirin. If you are taking aspirin for pain relief related to arthritis or other inflammatory conditions, it's best to take it one-half hour before you begin exercising for maximum pain relief.[1]

Another commonly-prescribed antiplatelet agent is Plavix". Although it thins the blood similarly to aspirin, it doesn't act as an anti-inflammatory or pain and fever reducer.

When taking Plavix", you can expect frequent blood work to monitor your blood count as well as liver enzymes. It is important to inform dentists and all health care providers that you are taking Plavix". Dental cleanings as well as other medical procedures may have to be put on hold until Plavix" had been stopped for at least seven days.

If you are taking Plavix", the only concern from an exercise standpoint is if you notice increased bruising or bleeding under your skin. If you see those changes, it is important to let your physician know about this. He or she may want to investigate this further and possibly make a medication or dosage change.

Effient" is an alternative to Plavix" that is commonly prescribed for those who require an antiplatelet agent and who are taking a proton-pump inhibitor such as Nexium" or Protonix". These medications are used for those suffering from acid reflux disease and to prevent ulcers. Studies indicate that when taking proton-pump inhibitors, the absorption of Plavix" is hindered, thus making it ineffective.[2] Effient", however, travels through a different metabolic pathway which does not affect this. Otherwise, the same precautions and considerations apply to both of these antiplatelet medications.

In terms of any exercise considerations, the only thing to really be aware of is any bruising you might experience. If you were to simply bump into an exercise machine, you might have a noticeable bruise to the affected extremity. As I had mentioned in the last chapter about a client of mine who had sustained a biceps strain, you could expect to see a deep discoloration at the site of the muscle strain, regardless of where the injury is. This is a typical side effect of medications like Effient˙ and Plavix˙. You should notify your doctor if bruising becomes so significant that it looks like you are dressed in military fatigues due to the abundant blotches of bruise marks.

ACE Inhibitors

ACE stands for *Angiotensin Converting Enzyme*. Angiotensin is a hormone that causes blood vessels to constrict, causing high blood pressure and strain on the heart. ACE is an enzyme that activates it. The goal of an ACE inhibitor is to prevent this enzyme from activating angiotensin. Use of ACE inhibitors results in dilated blood vessels, thus lowering blood pressure. It can also help prevent water retention. It is used to treat high blood pressure and/or heart failure. It prolongs survival of patients who've had an MI (myocardial infarction), and reduces the risk of MI and stroke in those with blood vessel disease. It can offer support for leaking heart valves.[1]

Examples of ACE inhibitors are Captopril˙, Enalapril˙, Quinipril˙ and Lisinopril˙. Chances are good if the name of the drug ends in "il," it's an ACE inhibitor. Possible side effects include dizziness, syncope (fainting), hypotension (low blood pressure), a frequent dry cough, a metallic taste in the mouth and hyperkalemia (high potassium in the blood).

Consider, with this medication, that you don't want to discontinue it abruptly, for a potential rebound effect. It would be a good idea to keep watch over your blood pressure, especially if you are feeling lightheaded. You may need to talk to your doctor about a dosage change.

In terms of exercise considerations, it's wise to rise slowly from a sitting or lying position to minimize lightheadedness and/or prevent fainting. Like other blood pressure medications, you may experience lightheadedness immediately after exercise, when your blood pressure tends to be lower. Inform your doctor if you become lightheaded after exercise. The fact that you are now exercising on a regular basis may warrant a dosage adjustment. Notify your doctor immediately if you were to faint. Be sure to take your ACE inhibitor before exercise to prevent your blood pressure from rising too high during your workout.

If you experience the side effect of a dry cough and it becomes bothersome, let your physician know; other options exist. Let your physician also know if you suffer from the metallic taste. In many cases, this symptom is improved in about eight to 10 weeks.

One other side effect worth mentioning is hyperkalemia. This risk can be minimized if you refrain from potassium salt substitutes, potassium supplements, potassium-sparing diuretics, and excessive potassium-rich foods such as bananas, orange juice, potatoes, or spinach.

Angiotensin Receptor Blockers

Angiotensin receptor blockers (ARB) are similar to ACE inhibitors. The main difference is that they block angiotensin through a different mechanism than ACE inhibitors. Examples of ARBs are Cozaar˙ and Diovan˙. ARBs tend to be prescribed for patients who suffer from the many side effects of ACE inhibitors, particularly the dry, nagging cough.

Many of the same exercise considerations for ACE inhibitors still apply to ARBs, including potential dizziness and fainting. Inform your doctor immediately if you were to faint. Like all blood pressure medications, be sure to take your ARB before exercise. This will prevent your blood pressure from rising too high during your workout. It is important to also mention that if you miss a dose, take it as soon as possible, unless the next dose is due within an hour.

Beta Blockers

When nervous, frightened or physically active, our bodies produce adrenalin. Adrenalin makes the heart beat stronger and faster, as well as constricting our blood vessels, causing a rise in blood pressure. Adrenalin works by latching onto structures called beta receptors on the muscle cells of the heart. Beta blockers prevent adrenalin from attaching to these receptors, which slows the heart rate and lowers the blood pressure.

In addition to lowering blood pressure, beta blockers reduce the contractility (strength) of the heart, which causes a slower and weaker beat. They are used to treat certain abnormal heart rhythms and heart failure, in addition to migraine headaches, glaucoma and tremors. Use of beta blockers has been shown to prolong survival of patients who have suffered a heart attack.[1]

Examples of beta blockers are metoprolol (Lopressor˙), Atenolol˙, Labetalol˙,and Coreg˙. There are beta-1 and beta-2 receptors, as well as alpha receptors. Certain beta blockers target both alpha and betas, whereas others block beta-1 and/or beta-2. For the most part, side effects are similar. Many of these drugs differ in their length of effectiveness. Toprol XL˙, for example, is an extended-release beta blocker.

The major side effects of beta blockers include a decreased heart rate, which could become too low if the dosage isn't right (i.e. under 50 bpm).

Hypotension is another possible side effect, with lightheadedness and fatigue accompanying it. Bronchospasm is another major side effect. This would be a narrowing of the airway, as a result of specific beta receptors being blocked. Because of this side effect, beta blockers are usually contraindicated in patients with chronic obstructive pulmonary disease (COPD) and asthma. Impotence may be an additional side effect. Usually decreasing the dosage may help. Cool extremities are another potential side effect, worth reporting to your physician.

An important thing to consider when taking this medication is to check your heart rate and blood pressure regularly. Unless you receive alternative orders from your physician, you should probably not take a dose of this medicine if your heart rate is less than 60 bpm and/or your systolic blood pressure (top number) is below 90 mmHg. Taking this medication will only decrease these numbers further, which can only increase negative side effects.

Additional points of consideration are to notify your doctor if you feel short of breath, dizzy or confused, or if your heart rate remains less than 60 bpm on a daily basis. This medicine should not be discontinued abruptly. You need to gradually taper the dose over a two-week period, in order to prevent a rebound angina. Take this medicine with food for increased absorption.

From an exercise standpoint, be aware that your aerobic exercise prescription will vary if you are taking a beta blocker. Not only will your resting heart rate be decreased, your exercise heart rate will also be reduced. When performing aerobic exercise, you might aim to get your target heart rate within a range of 60-85% of your age-predicted maximum heart rate. Let's say the value is 120-145 bpm.

If you are not taking a beta blocker, you may comfortably exercise in this range. However, if you are taking this medication, it's not uncommon that you may reach only 90-100 bpm, with the same effort level. If you weren't aware of this, you might push harder than necessary to get to your target heart rate, which could be dangerous.

For those who suffer from angina, you can expect an increase in exercise capacity with a beta blocker. For those without angina, exercise capacity may be decreased or there may be no change with a beta blocker on board.

Calcium Channel Blockers

Calcium ions help the heart and blood vessels to work effectively. The goal of calcium channel blockers is to partially prevent calcium from doing this job. Preventing the heart and blood vessels from doing their most energetic work relaxes the muscles in the walls of arteries, allowing arteries to open wider. This results in a lowered blood pressure and an improved blood supply to the heart. Calcium channel blockers also relax the heart muscle. All of these effects allow the heart to effectively function with a reduced blood supply.

Calcium channel blockers are used to lower blood pressure, control angina, treat certain cardiac arrhythmias, prevent vascular spasms after brain hemorrhage, and help prevent migraines. Some of the more commonly prescribed calcium channel blockers are Norvasc˙ and Cardizem˙. Side effects include lightheadedness, especially when rising from a lying or sitting position, possible abdominal discomfort or loss of appetite, and possible hypotension and/or prolonged heart rate of less than 60 bpm (bradycardia).

With calcium channel blockers, it is important to check your pulse before administering. The medication may need to be held back if your resting heart rate is less than 60 bpm. It is also important to routinely check your blood pressure. You would want to hold the medication if your systolic blood pressure is <90 mmHg. If experiencing dizziness, in addition to notifying your physician, you should avoid hazardous activities until the issue has been resolved. You also want to inform your physician if you experience shortness of breath or palpitations. This is another medicine that should not be stopped abruptly.

From an exercise perspective, you may experience a decreased heart rate and blood pressure. Let your physician know if you feel lightheaded. This is especially possible after exercise when your blood pressure tends to be lower. If you suffer from angina, you can expect an increase in exercise capacity; meaning you will be able to exercise harder and longer. If you do not suffer from angina, calcium channel blockers should not affect your exercise capacity.

As you will learn in the next chapter, proper nutrition is essential to productive workouts. If you suffer from the side effects of abdominal discomfort or a loss of appetite, notify your physician so you both can explore alternatives. You don't want your workouts or recovery period to be hindered because of poor nutrition.

Diuretics

Diuretics remove fluid from the body by increasing urination. They are used to treat hypertension, fluid retention (related to heart failure, kidney failure, cirrhosis, or CHF), some forms of kidney disease, Meniere's disease (inner ear), diabetes, and to help prevent calcium-based kidney stones. In a nutshell, diuretics cause the kidneys to excrete unnecessary water and salt from the body through the urine.

There are several types of diuretics. Loop diuretics tend to be the strongest form, preventing the reabsorption of sodium and chloride by the intestines. As a result, water, in addition to electrolytes such as potassium and magnesium, are removed from the body. Furosemide (Lasix˚) is the most common loop diuretic.

A second type is a thiazide diuretic. The most common one is Hydrochlorothiazide˚ (HCTZ˚). As opposed to loop diuretics, thiazide diuretics act on a different part of the intestine. The end result is similar, however, with excretion of sodium, chloride, potassium and water. Metolazone˚ is another thiazide diuretic frequently prescribed. Zaroxolyn˚ is an extended-release form.

Diamox˚ (Acetazolamide) is a diuretic with similar properties to loop and thiazide diuretics in that it prevents reabsorption of water, sodium and potassium. It inhibits enzyme activity in an area of the kidneys, as opposed to areas of the intestines as in loop and thiazide diuretics.

A third type is a potassium-sparing diuretic. Aldactone˚ and Triamterene˚ are examples. This particular diuretic competes with the hormone aldosterone, at receptor sites located in the intestine. Aldosterone is a hormone produced at the kidney, which causes salt and water retention. This medication will have the opposite effect, in which water, sodium and chloride are excreted. It differs from the other forms of diuretics in that potassium and phosphates are retained.

Potential side effects of potassium-sparing diuretics are hyperkalemia (high potassium in the blood), GI bleeding, diarrhea, headaches, cramping, and gynocomastia (breast enlargement in males). With these drugs, you'll need to avoid foods high in potassium such as bananas, oranges and salt substitutes. You should notify your doctor if you develop cramping, diarrhea, headaches, gynocomastia or lethargy.

Many potential side effects of loop and thiazide diuretics tend to be similar to those for Diamox˚. All three would put you at risk for hypokalemia, hyperglycemia, cramps, fatigue and photosensitivity to light. Be sure to use sunscreen when going outdoors, due to photosensitivity.

With hyperglycemia, you may experience increased thirst, headaches, difficulty concentrating, blurred vision, frequent urination, and fatigue. If you do experience any of these effects, you should not hesitate to check your blood sugar. Your blood sugar shouldn't be greater than 140mg/dL after meals if you do not have diabetes. If you do have diabetes, your blood sugar should range between 80 and 180 mg/dL before exercise. Depending on how low your blood sugar gets after exercise, you may need to adjust your glucose-lowering medications or your carbohydrate intake, based on your doctor's recommendations. You should notify your doctor if your blood sugars are ranging greater than 200mg/dL or less than 70mg/dL, regardless of whether it is before or after exercise.

Unlike potassium-sparing diuretics, with both loop and thiazides you'll want to keep potassium-rich foods in your diet. The greatest concern with hypokalemia is developing potentially fatal heart arrhythmias. Depending on the dosage of your loop or thiazide diuretics, as well as the potassium levels in your blood, a potassium supplement may be prescribed by your doctor. Be sure to discuss with your doctor whether a potassium supplement would be right for you. With all diuretics, it's best to take them in the morning, to prevent losing sleep related to frequent urination.

With regard to exercise, diuretics should not affect an exercise capacity except potentially in CHF patients. Blood pressure may be lower at rest and after exercise, but no direct effect with exercise is expected. Notify your doctor if experiencing dizziness or fainting. Chances are greater of experiencing this after exercise, when blood pressure tends to be lower. If you tend to sweat a lot during exercise, your risk for dehydration increases, especially when taking diuretics. Be aware of cramps and excessive tiredness, which are signs of dehydration and can be caused by loop and thiazide diuretics. Notify your doctor if you experience these side effects.

<u>Lipid-lowering Agents</u>

Lipid- or cholesterol-lowering agents fall into three categories. There are HMG-CoA reductase inhibitors, which are drugs that inhibit or prevent an enzyme from making cholesterol. Lipitor˙ (atorvastatin) and Zocor˙ (simvastatin) are examples. They tend to be recognized as "statins." Side effects include muscle pain and tenderness, liver dysfunction, rhabdomyolysis (a serious disorder in which muscle cells are broken down), and lens opacities, requiring annual eye exams .[1] The most common of these side effects tend to be the muscle pain and tenderness.

From an exercise standpoint, this could significantly limit your exercise tolerance. For most, it is bearable. If you are one of the unlucky ones to be bothered by this, inform your physician. There may be other options.

A second type of lipid-lowering agent is a bile acid sequestrant. This is a drug that reduces the amount of bile acid our bodies produce. Decreased bile acid results in lower cholesterol. Questran˙ is one example. Side effects include muscle and/or joint pain, possible deficiency of vitamins A, D and K, and increased risk of bleeding. You will need to be alert for blood in urine or stool, which would require medical attention. Be sure to take this medication at a different time from other medications or food for maximal absorption.

Similar to "statins," exercise should not be affected by this medication. However, if you experience muscle or joint pain that is significantly compromising exercise, notify your physician.

The last type of lipid-lowering drug is a folic acid derivative. This drug inhibits the manufacturing of LDL and VLDL, which make triglycerides. Tricor˙ is an example of this drug. Possible side effects include dysrhythmia, muscle pain, fatigue, decreased urine output, potential blood in the urine, and impotence. It would be wise to let your doctor know if you experience any of these side effects.

Similarly to the other types of lipid-lowering drugs, muscle or joint pain is a potential side effect. Be sure to let your doctor know if muscle discomfort is limiting your ability to exercise. Keep in mind that with all of these drugs, most people tolerate exercise just fine.

<u>Nitrates</u>

Nitrates are drugs that dilate (widen) the arteries in the heart, which improves blood flow to the heart muscle. Nitrates also dilate the veins, so that the heart does not have to beat as strongly to move blood along. Nitrates also have a mild anti-clotting effect. Nitrates are used to reduce or stop angina attacks.

Nitroglycerin is the most common nitrate prescribed. There are many different forms through which the medication can be administered. It can be given through a patch (Nitro-dur˙), ointment (Nitro-bid˙), spray (Nitrolingual spray˙), and pills; some of which are chewed, swallowed or dissolved under the tongue. Imdur˙ is an example of a longer-acting form of nitroglycerin in pill form.

With longer-acting forms of nitroglycerin (i.e. Imdur˙, Nitro-dur˙), they are not meant to relieve acute chest pain (angina). Their job is to prevent it. To relieve angina during an acute attack, the fast-acting forms, such as sublingual nitroglycerin, are often prescribed. The idea is to take one sublingual tab at the onset of chest pain. If there is no relief after five minutes, take another. If there is no relief after another five minutes, take another tab. If there is no relief after three tabs of nitroglycerin in 15 minutes, you must seek immediate medical attention.

Side effects of nitrates include headache, lightheadedness, postural hypotension and possible elevated heart rate. Important to remember with nitroglycerin (particularly the sublingual form) is to carry it with you at all times. You should keep the tablets in a moisture-proof, dark container; away from light. You should have the prescription renewed after one year if the bottle is unopened; six months if opened.

It is important that you do not take nitroglycerin if you have taken the medication Viagra`, due to a potentially fatal drop in blood pressure. With lightheadedness as a potential side effect, be sure to remain seated when taking this medication.

With exercise, nitrates may give you an increased heart rate, or it may remain unchanged. Blood pressure may be lower or remain unchanged with exercise. For those with angina, nitrates will increase their exercise capacity. I have seen this firsthand, where my client's exercise capacity was limited due to chest pain. He is a musician who takes weekly trips into New York City from Connecticut. Especially during the winter months when he is breathing in the cold outdoor air, he would have great difficulty walking to his rehearsals. For those unfamiliar with New York City, walking is the primary mode of transportation. This client expressed his concern to me that he was unsure if he'd be able to perform in the annual Holiday concert, due to his angina while walking. I could understand his concern, for his maximum speed on the treadmill was barely two miles an hour.

Although sublingual nitroglycerin was one of his prescribed medications, he was never instructed to take the medication prophylactically before exercise. In other words, he knew to take the medicine if he experienced chest pain. He was not aware that he could potentially take it before exercise, to *prevent* the occurrence of chest pain. Before introducing the idea to him, I checked with his cardiologist to ensure that it was acceptable to take nitroglycerin *before* exercise. His cardiologist was fine with the idea of using the medication in this manner. Sure enough, taking nitroglycerin prior to exercise increased his exercise capacity to the point where he was able to walk at 2.3 miles per hour with a 2% incline on the treadmill! He was able to nearly double his duration of exercise, as well. More importantly, he was able to handle the long walks in New York City on those cold, wintery evenings as he travelled to his rehearsals. It was a pleasure not only to see his progress in cardiac rehab, but his performance in that Holiday concert as well.

If you have a prescription from your doctor for sublingual nitroglycerin to take as needed, it may be advantageous to take it prophylactically immediately before exercise or sexual activity. If you don't have a prescription for nitroglycerin, and your exercise capacity is limited by angina, it would be wise to discuss this with your physician.

Although not a nitrate, Renexa` is a more recent addition to the list of antianginal medications that should be addressed. It is prescribed to help relieve symptoms of angina when patients are not responding adequately to other antianginal drugs. The exact way in which it relieves angina symptoms is unknown. Nevertheless, it has antianginal and anti-ischemic effects that do not depend on heart rate or blood pressure. Studies have shown a significant reduction in angina attacks and fewer nitroglycerin requirements than the placebo.[3] Those with certain specific EKG abnormalities, impaired liver, or who are on medications such as Cardizem˙ and certain antibiotics, should avoid Renexa˙. Neither grapefruit nor grapefruit juice should be consumed if on this medication. Notify your physician if you experience palpitations or fainting spells while using it. Otherwise, it may be helpful in enabling an individual with chronic, stable angina to work at a greater capacity without the same level of discomfort.

Exercise considerations: Your heart rate may be slightly elevated, but it should not be of any significance. Your blood pressure may be lower. As a result, be aware of any lightheadedness and be sure to remain in a seated position when administering nitroglycerin. When chest pain or lightheadedness subsides, it should be safe to resume exercise. On a scale of one to four, with four being the maximum chest pain experienced and one being the least, you should not have chest pain greater than a two. Beyond a two on this pain scale, be sure to take a nitroglycerin dose as ordered according to protocol (one dose every five minutes for a maximum of three doses. After the third dose, if chest pain is still present, call 911). If you have known chest pain with exertion, discuss taking nitroglycerin *before* exercise to increase your exercise capacity.

Respiratory Agents

Although respiratory agents don't fall into the category of cardiac medications, enough people suffer from asthma, emphysema and COPD that these conditions often result in exercise limitations. After all, if you can't breathe, you're not going to make it very far on the treadmill. Since medications to deal with these conditions are commonly prescribed, it's worth mentioning the most common ones.

There are many types of drugs in several categories under the heading: respiratory agents. There are steroidal anti-inflammatory agents, such as Flovent˙ and Advair Discus˙, which are commonly prescribed to those suffering from asthma. There are anticholinergics, such as Atrovent˙, which allows bronchial smooth muscle to relax, opening up the airway. This is given to those with COPD to prevent bronchospasm (narrowing of the airway).

Another type of respiratory agent is a sympathomimetic, also known as a beta-2 receptor agonist. If you recall our discussion with beta blockers, I had mentioned there are beta-1 and beta-2 receptors. I also mentioned that a possible side effect with beta blockers is bronchoconstriction, whereby the airway is narrowed. The job of sympathomimetics (i.e. Albuterol˙) is to help the beta-2 receptors, not block them. The end result is that the airway is opened wide, allowing easier breathing. This is commonly used to prevent exercise-induced asthma, as well as bronchitis, emphysema or other reversible airway obstruction.

A final type of respiratory agent is a xanthine derivative. An example is a drug called Theophyline˙. It is a spasmolyte, which simply relaxes the smooth muscle of the respiratory system. It is used for bronchospasm of COPD, bronchial asthma and chronic bronchitis. It is not commonly prescribed to those with heart disease, due to the many potential negative cardiovascular side effects.

The important thing to note about respiratory agents from an exercise standpoint is that they can increase exercise capacity in those limited by bronchospasm, in which a person suddenly becomes short of breath due to a narrowing of the airway. This can be due to asthma, medications such as beta blockers or an allergen.

These respiratory agents act as performance-enhancers, enabling sufferers to exercise harder and for a longer period of time, without feeling so short of breath. It is crucial for those suffering from bronchospasms to be compliant with their medication. Simply missing a dose can allow breathing difficulties to resume. Just as it is important to be compliant with exercise in order to reap the numerous benefits, medication compliance is no less important. For those not limited by bronchospasm, exercise capacity will remain unchanged.

Anti-diabetic Agents

There are several types of drugs that fit under the category of anti-diabetic agents. These are medications that help correct abnormal blood glucose levels. Depending on the type of drug, we will know how it works in the body to lower blood glucose levels.

One type of anti-diabetic drug is a *biguanide*, a drug that decreases glucose production in the liver and increases tissue sensitivity to insulin. So, if your pancreas still produces some insulin, what little insulin it does produce will be more effective. An example of a biguanide is Glucophage˙. It comes in pill form and should be taken with food.

Another commonly prescribed anti-diabetic agent is a *sulfonylurea*. This is a drug that stimulates beta cells in the pancreas to produce more insulin. It may improve insulin-binding to insulin receptors as well. Similar to biguanides, sulfonylureas are available in pill form. Glipizide˙, Glyburide˙ and Amaryl˙ are examples.

Another anti-diabetic agent is a *thiazolidinedione*, a type of drug that increases insulin sensitivity. This will increase the effectiveness of what little insulin our pancreas does make. An example of this type is Actos˙. Avandia˙ was a frequently prescribed type that was recalled due to the serious risk of heart attacks, strokes, CHF and increased incidence of osteoporosis. A study published in the *New England Journal of Medicine* in May 2007 showed that in 42 previous studies involving 1400 patients taking Avandia˙, users suffered a significant 43% more heart attacks than those taking the placebo.[4]

For the three types of anti-diabetic agents mentioned, there are similarities worth mentioning. All three types of drugs are meant for those with type II diabetes, where the pancreas still produces some insulin. (In type I diabetes, the pancreas doesn't really produce any at all, making these drugs ineffective.)

Another similarity is that all three of these types of medications will stress the liver and kidneys. As a result, frequent blood work is necessary. You need to be sure to check your blood sugar periodically, to monitor the effectiveness of your dosage as well as to monitor your diet. It's important to be compliant with your medications, as well as to stick to your diet. Dietary considerations would be following a diet high in fiber and low in sugar. Consuming small frequent meals helps ensure you aren't taking in too many grams of sugar with each meal. Consuming some protein and fiber with each meal can help stabilize your blood sugar. In the next chapter, you will find guidelines along with sample diets that can be applied and/or modified for those with diabetes.

There is another type of anti-diabetic medication that is used in type II diabetes, called Byetta˙. It basically mimics natural physiology for self-regulating glycemic control. It can be used in conjunction with any of the three previously-described types of agents, although it's not commonly prescribed. It's available only in subcutaneous injection form where you would administer a needle within the fat layer under your skin. Gastrointestinal side effects can be particularly bothersome.

The most commonly prescribed anti-diabetic agent, especially for type I diabetes, is insulin. It also happens to be the most dangerous. In addition to being a drug, insulin is a hormone, manufactured by beta cells in the pancreas. Insulin is actually the most anabolic (muscle building) hormone in our body;

more anabolic than testosterone! It helps shuttle amino acids into our muscle tissue, which explains the anabolism.[5] It also helps shuttle glucose out of the blood and into our body's tissues. This helps regulate a normal blood glucose level. For those with type I diabetes, the pancreas is not making insulin, so the solution is to administer insulin from outside the body to inside. Insulin is usually administered through a subcutaneous injection, to an area with some body fat, such as our thigh, abdomen, or upper arm.

There are several different types of insulin, differentiated by the length of time it takes to become effective to how long it stays effective. For example, Humalog* is a human form of insulin that takes effect in 15 minutes and lasts for three to five hours. Humalin R* is a regular insulin that takes effect in 30-60 minutes, and lasts for five to seven hours. Lantus* is a slow-acting form taking effect in one to two hours and lasting 24 hours. There are also mixtures available, which are combinations of fast and slower-acting insulin.

With whatever form of insulin you use, you need to closely monitor your blood sugar and take the correct dosage. Keep in mind that none of these drugs cure diabetes; they can only control it. You should keep insulin and emergency equipment with you at all times. Have simple sugars such as candy or glucose tablets present and available to you, in case of hypoglycemia. Symptoms of hypoglycemia include sweating, weakness, dizziness, chills, confusion, headaches, nausea, rapid pulse, slurred speech, anxiety, tremors, hunger, fatigue, and staggered gait. Wearing an emergency identification bracelet as a diabetic would be wise. Signs of hyperglycemia (high blood sugar) include fruity breath, warm and dry skin, fatigue, and frequent urination. If you're finding it very difficult to keep your blood sugar in an acceptable range, you should work closely with an endocrinologist and a diabetes educator/nutritionist as well.

The reason I am giving so much attention to insulin in this chapter is that exercise has a definite effect on blood sugar. Whether or not we have diabetes, exercise does a great job of decreasing blood sugar, as well as increasing the body's sensitivity to insulin, which helps further reduce blood sugar.

It is not uncommon for those on anti-diabetic medication to eventually need a reduction in dosage, due to the effects of exercise. In some cases, I've seen individuals taken off anti-diabetic medications, simply because their blood sugars became so well-controlled through diet and exercise! How great would it be if you didn't have to take those injections every day?

When first starting an exercise program (or resuming after a long break), it would be wise to check your blood sugar before, during and after exercise. This will help you learn how exercise and diet affect your glucose levels. You will be able to learn how many carbohydrates you need and how much insulin will be required. You have to be very responsible and on top of your own care. With diabetes, especially with insulin, there is little room for error.

The importance of medication compliance

I cannot bring this chapter to a close without emphasizing the significance of medication compliance. Doctors prescribe medications for a reason. If you're not sure why, it is your right and obligation to ask and to find out why you have been prescribed each and every medication that you are taking. How can you expect to take your medications as prescribed if you're not sure what you're putting into your body and why?

You also want to be aware of potential side effects. If you experience such reactions, discuss this with your doctor. Some of these side effects may be harmful if prolonged. If you are uncertain about how and when to take a certain medication, ask your doctor or your pharmacist. A 2012 study showed that out of 851 heart patients, just over half do not take their medications correctly, even if pharmacists intervened through counseling, medication reconciliation and telephone follow-up after hospital discharge.[6]

If you have difficulty remembering to take a medication at a certain time, consider purchasing a pill box that is labeled for seven days a week at four different times of day: "Morning," "Noon," "Evening," and "Bedtime." It comes in particularly handy when traveling. I use one when traveling to national-level bodybuilding contests, where I need to keep luggage light. It does not do me any good to transport 14 bottles of vitamins, minerals and other supplements when I'm trying to make the luggage weight limit at the airport!

Be sure to keep a list of your medications in your wallet or in another easily accessible location. If there is a medical emergency and you become unresponsive, it can be vital that first responders know what medications you are currently taking.* At the very least, you will have a quick reference if asked what medications you take.

If cost is an issue with certain medications, discuss this with your physician. Physicians often can provide free samples, discount coupons, or can switch you to a generic brand or less-expensive alternative. Your doctor needs to be your teammate and partner. He or she can be of no help if there is a lack of communication. With medication compliance and a good working relationship

---

* If you do not already have a medication history sheet, a handy sheet that you could use for this purpose is available for you in the Appendix. If this is a library book, of course you will want to photocopy the sheet and not write in the book. You have my permission to photocopy that page.

between doctor and patient, you can expect a greater likelihood of optimal health.

Chapter 13

*Diet & Nutrition**

Mike was 44 years old when he suffered his heart attack five years ago. He had a 100% blockage of his left anterior descending artery, which caused symptoms while he was vacationing in Puerto Rico. This resulted in his having to get an angioplasty with two stents.

Nutrition played a role as one of the factors in his heart event. After his heart attack, Mike was forced to consider what changes he needed to make to avoid another attack:

> *Nutrition was another big concern for me* [in addition to exercise]. *Prior to my heart attack, I was aware that my cholesterol was high despite eating a relatively low-fat diet. I would look at labels and try to pick foods lower in saturated fat, in particular.*
>
> *Looking back, I realize I ate a lot of frozen dinners and snacked on a lot of chips. Despite coming from the health food section of the stores, they came with a lot of fat and preservatives.*
>
> *I also had the habit of "letting myself go" several times a week where I would eat anything – ice cream, fried eggs, etcetera. Now that I'm back at home, how do I eat to prevent another attack?*

Mike began a planned exercise program through the cardiac rehab center, availing himself of the reeducation in nutrition that it offered. As he explains:

> *Regarding nutrition, cardiac rehab has educated me on how to structure my diet both for heart health and exercise performance. I've increased my consumption of fruits, vegetables and whole grains, while cutting out excess simple sugars, fried foods and red meat. I've learned healthy alternatives to the unhealthy snacks I'd binged on for so many years. I now have structure in my diet, which has given me more structure in my life in general.*

---

* I want to thank Jillian DiViesta, RD, PA-C, dietitian and PA (physician assistant) for reviewing this chapter.

You may read Mike's story in its entirety in his own words in the Appendix at the end of this book.

Nutrition Basics

After understanding the benefits of exercise, and how to put together the workout program that your body and your heart need, understanding diet and nutrition is key to your heart health. With all of the fad diets that exist, along with contradictions as to which foods are "good" or "bad," it's no wonder a majority of people are left confused or misguided. As you read on, my goal is to help clear up that confusion for you.

Nutrition is the science of food; it involves learning the various nutrients that are necessary for optimal health, as well as *how much* and *what kinds* of foods are required to achieve beneficial results, such as growth and development, proper cellular functioning, disease prevention, health maintenance and energy. By learning the various nutrients, how the body uses them and how we can use them for optimum health, you will possess a great power. As the saying goes, "knowledge is power." Whether your goal is weight loss, weight gain, weight maintenance, having more energy, or blood sugar control, this chapter on nutrition and diet will guide you along the right path. (If you consider yourself knowledgeable in these areas, you might still find this chapter to be a useful review.)

There are three basic nutrients, known as macronutrients:

- protein
- carbohydrates
- fat

These are the essential nutrients to the healthy diet. Although not recognized as a macronutrient, water is an additional essential nutrient that must be present in your diet. It should be considered the king of nutrients simply because it's the major component of our body. It makes up 72% of our muscles. The importance of water cannot be overemphasized. *(See a further discussion of water below).*

Other nutrients are called micronutrients. The four micronutrients are:

- vitamins
- mineral
- essential amino acids
- essential fatty acids

Let's talk about each macronutrient and micronutrient in greater detail below.

Protein

Protein is made up of amino acids, which are the building blocks of our body's tissues. Your hair, skin, nails and muscle tissue are examples. Proteins are classified as either complete or incomplete. Complete proteins are foods that contain all of the essential amino acids necessary to produce *usable protein*. This means that the body will have what it needs for proper repair, recovery and growth. Examples of complete protein foods are eggs, meat, fish and milk. In contrast, incomplete proteins are foods that do not contain all of the essential amino acids and thus need to be combined with other foods to be complete. Examples are bread, rice, beans and nuts, and examples of combinations would be rice with beans, cereal with milk, and whole wheat bread with all-natural peanut butter.

Protein is an important part of your diet. It is vital to get a variety of protein sources to ensure you are getting all of the essential amino acids.

The recommended dietary allowance (RDA) of protein in the average diet is 0.8-1 gm/kg of bodyweight (2.2lbs) per day.[1,2] For a 150-pound individual, this would equate to about 68 grams of protein per day. Although this may be adequate for sedentary individuals, those who are exercising regularly can benefit from greater amounts. For athletes, in particular, there is a need for additional amino acids in the diet.[2]

As regular exercisers, we should consider ourselves athletes because in reality, we are. We are exercising for 30 to 60 minutes most days of the week, doing a combination of resistance training and cardiovascular exercise. This justifies the need for more protein in our diet. In order to get enough of the necessary amino acids to repair muscle breakdown and aid in muscle recovery and growth, taking in closer to 1 gram of protein per pound of bodyweight (150 grams for that 150-pound individual) may be more appropriate.

Drinking adequate amounts of water will help protect your kidneys from any potential stress caused by increased protein in your diet. Consuming enough calcium in the diet and/or supplementing additional calcium may help prevent any potential deficiencies related to a higher-protein diet, although studies have yet to prove this. What has been studied is that protein and calcium appear to act synergistically on bone if both are present in adequate quantities. But when calcium intake is low, protein may seem effectively antagonistic toward bone.[3] In this case, it makes sense to increase your consumption of dietary calcium (milk, yogurt, salmon, almonds, broccoli, spinach, etc.) as opposed to reducing your protein intake, which wouldn't be helpful to exercising muscles or bone.

Those who may need to limit their protein are those with any preexisting kidney disease or those with diabetes. These people are at an increased risk of renal problems related to poorly controlled blood sugar. Excess protein will cause additional stress to their kidneys, which may be problematic. These people will need to discuss with their endocrinologist or urologist what a safe maximum daily amount of protein would be.

Although 1 gram of protein per pound of bodyweight per day may seem excessive, if you divide the total into four to six small meals per day, you may be surprised at how realistic and achievable this is. This could equate to anywhere from 20 to 50 grams of protein per meal for most individuals, depending on bodyweight and number of meals chosen to eat per day. Such meal frequency will be satiating and meet your protein needs.

What about protein supplements? There are numerous products on the market, from protein shakes, bars, cookies, ice cream and brownies, to juices, that provide additional protein in the diet. There are three types of protein that are typically used in these protein supplements: milk, egg, and soy.

Milk proteins come in three forms: whey, milk protein concentrate, and calcium caseinate. Whey has gained the most popularity, being that it is easily digested, high in branched chain amino acids (BCAAs), and could help support proper immune function.[4,5,6] In simple terms, BCAAs are three amino acids (leucine, isoleucine and valine) which are especially important for muscle repair, recovery and growth.

In choosing a protein supplement, athletes in particular will want a protein high in BCAAs. Whey protein isolate and whey protein concentrate are the most popular wheys on the market. Whey isolate is the purest of the two, with increased bioavailability. But it is also the most expensive. It is 100% lactose free, so for those who are intolerant to lactose, whey protein isolate is the way to go.

Milk protein concentrate and calcium caseinate are the other two milk derivatives. They digest more slowly than whey, which may fill you up more. Egg protein is usually listed as egg albumen under the list of ingredients of an egg protein supplement. Most protein supplements will have a mixture of milk and egg proteins.

Soy protein, a vegetable source of protein, takes the longest to digest. Research has shown that soy protein can help lower serum cholesterol in some individuals. For those with heart disease and taking cholesterol-lowering medications, soy may be your best choice. Examples of soy foods are tofu, soybeans, veggie burgers, soy milk and soy nuts.

There have been concerns in recent years that high amounts of phytoestrogens like soy-based isoflavone compounds may have negative health consequences such as possibly promoting breast and uterine cancers. Phytoestrogens are estrogen-like compounds found in plants. Recent studies from 2011 and 2012 have shown no adverse effects of soy foods on breast cancer prognosis.[7,8] For those wishing to remain conservative, one to three servings of soy per day (1 serving = ½ cup) can be considered a moderate amount and generally safe.

Keep in mind that protein supplements are just that, *supplements*. A supplement is something that is added to help meet your requirements. It's not meant to be a substitute for food. However, if you aim for about one gram of protein per pound of bodyweight per day, it may be difficult to meet that requirement with food alone. For those needing to watch cholesterol levels, getting the majority of protein through high-cholesterol meats may not be the best way to go. But by having a meal or two with fish, meat or poultry, one or two protein shakes or another kind of protein supplement, and maybe a meal of rice and beans, for example, you can easily meet your daily protein requirements without a high intake of cholesterol.

Carbohydrates

Carbohydrates are the body's main and most easily accessible source of energy. All carbohydrates are sugars. There is blood sugar, fruit sugar, table sugar, milk sugar, malt sugar, starch, cellulose and glycogen. Once ingested, all carbohydrates will convert into glucose.

The glycemic index is a measurement of how quickly carbohydrates are metabolized. Carbohydrates that convert quickly into glucose are known as high glycemic index (GI) carbohydrates. Examples are processed sugar, cereals and carrots.

Carbohydrates with a low GI are metabolized over a period of time, giving a more sustained release of energy. Examples are milk, yogurt, lentils and cold weather fruits (i.e., apples, peaches, pears, grapes); moderate GI foods are tropical fruits, oats and sucrose.

Many of the recent fad diets suggest that you limit the high glycemic carbohydrates because of the immediate rise in blood sugar after consuming such foods. This rise in blood sugar causes the pancreas to release more insulin, which can cause a heightened ability to store body fat. Couple that with the quick drop in blood sugar from excess insulin production, and the appetite is stimulated, leaving you feeling hungrier with intense cravings. (I will discuss later in the chapter whether high glycemic carbohydrates can and should be labeled as "bad" carbohydrates, and what types should be consumed and what types should be limited).

In addition to providing the body's most efficient energy source, carbohydrates serve other important functions such as providing the main source of energy that fuels the functioning of the brain and muscles. For those deprived of carbohydrates, muscle will be broken down and utilized as energy to support brain function. This is known as ketosis.

Carbohydrates have a protein-sparing effect. Without adequate consumption of carbohydrates, protein can be used as energy. The problem with this, as previously discussed, is that protein is needed for tissue repair, recovery and growth. If protein is being used for energy because you lack carbohydrates in your diet, the amino acids will not be available for tissue repair, recovery and growth.

Another function of carbohydrates is providing your body with ample supplies of glycogen, which is the carbohydrate stored in muscle. The carbohydrates stored in muscle in the form of glycogen are what enable us to exercise for long periods of time.

Fiber

A type of carbohydrate that is particularly vital is fiber. There are two kinds of fiber: soluble and insoluble.

Soluble fiber is a fiber that absorbs water. Examples are oats, dried beans and peas, nuts, flax seeds, fruits and vegetables. Examples of fruits are peaches, plums, apples, pears, blueberries and prunes. Examples of vegetables are Brussels sprouts, sweet potatoes, asparagus, turnips, beets, broccoli, onions and green peppers. Soluble fiber binds with fatty acids to clear from the gut, in turn lowering cholesterol. It also prolongs stomach emptying time so sugar is released and absorbed more slowly. Soluble fiber has been shown to lower both total and LDL (bad) cholesterol. It also helps regulate blood sugar, especially important for those with or at risk for diabetes.

Insoluble fiber helps bulk stool, moving it through the intestine, promoting regular bowel movements, preventing constipation. It also helps reduce the risk of colon cancer. Sources of insoluble fiber include dark green leafy vegetables, green beans, whole wheat, fruit skins, root vegetable skins, nuts and seeds.

Most fiber foods contain a mixture of both soluble and insoluble fiber. No recommended intake of each separate fiber exists. But for optimum health, the Academy of Nutrition and Dietetics recommends a minimum of 20-35gm per day. Although this may seem difficult to meet, consuming small meals every three to four hours and having a little fiber with each of those meals can help you reach this goal and not seem overwhelming. It is important to note that if you are nowhere near the recommended value per day, increase your consumption slowly to prevent gas and upset stomach.

Fat

The last of the macronutrients is fat. Fat provides the major source of energy, serves to cushion and protect major organs, and acts as an insulator, holding on to body heat to protect you against the cold.

Fat molecules differ in composition and can be classified as being saturated, unsaturated or polyunsaturated.

Saturated fat is found in foods such as beef, lamb, pork, chicken, shellfish, egg yolks, cheese, milk, butter, chocolate, lard and vegetable shortening. The more saturated the fat, the more likely it is to stay in the body, clogging arteries and increasing the risk of heart disease and stroke. Diets high in saturated fat can elevate blood cholesterol levels, promoting the formation of plaque in our arteries. The American Heart Association recommends no more than 10% of your total caloric intake be composed of saturated fat. In order to reduce your risk of heart disease, the guidelines are stricter with less than 7% of your total caloric intake being composed of saturated fat.

A type of fat similar to saturated fat that is important to mention is trans fat. Trans fats are fatty acids created in an industrial process that makes liquid vegetable oils more solid by adding hydrogen to them. They can be identified in the ingredients listing on food labels by the name *partially hydrogenated oils*. They are added to foods because they provide a desirable taste and texture. They are mainly found in fried foods and baked goods. Examples are French fries, cookies, cakes, doughnuts, crackers, margarine sticks and shortenings. Trans fats increase LDL and lower HDL cholesterol levels. As such, consuming them increases your risk for heart disease, stroke and diabetes. The American Heart Association recommends limiting trans fats to less than 1% of your total caloric intake or less than 2 grams per day. Some trans fats occur naturally in some meat and dairy products, including beef, lamb and butterfat. It has not yet been determined if naturally-occurring trans fats pose the same health risks as industrially manufactured sources. Since most of us probably consume naturally occurring trans fats, there's no place for industrially manufactured trans fats in your diet.

Unsaturated fat tends to be liquid at room temperature. However, you will see there are exceptions. Examples of unsaturated fat are olives, olive oil, peanuts, peanut oil, peanut butter and avocados. This fat is considered more favorable in the diet.

Monounsaturated fat is the most neutral of fats in that it doesn't affect your cholesterol like some other fats do. Monounsaturated fat is found in foods such as olive oil, macadamia nuts and canola oil. I would place them in the category of "good" fat; they should make up a greater percentage of your daily fat intake.

Polyunsaturated fat is yet another type of fat. Polyunsaturated fat contains essential fatty acids, which must be present in the diet because the body doesn't manufacture them. Of particular importance are omega-3 and omega-6 fatty acids. Many health benefits have been recognized related to increased consumption of omega-3 fatty acids. They have been shown to increase HDL (good) cholesterol, which indirectly lowers LDL (bad) cholesterol. Omega-3 fatty acids have also been shown to contain blood-thinning properties.[9] This may be especially beneficial for people with heart disease. Those on blood-thinning medications such as Plavix° and Coumadin° should use caution when considering supplementing with additional omega-3 fatty acids. This is generally not of concern with food sources of omega-3s. Up to 3 grams per day of omega-3 fatty acids are generally recognized as safe. Significantly higher doses may increase your risk for a hemorrhagic stroke. If you have any doubt about their safety and are taking potent blood-thinning medications, check with your cardiologist.

Omega-3 fatty acids also have an anti-inflammatory effect. Current research suggests that those suffering from rheumatoid arthritis who consume adequate omega-3 fatty acids have less pain compared to those taking non-steroidal anti-inflammatory drugs such as ibuprofen.[10]

Omega-6 fatty acids, on the other hand, may need to be consumed with a little more care. Although omega-6 fatty acids have similar health benefits, too much omega-6s with not enough omega-3s can actually cause an increase in LDL with a decrease in HDL cholesterol, essentially having a reverse effect! An effective ratio may be in the neighborhood of 6:1 omega-3s:omega-6s.[11] Keep in mind that omega-6s do have their health benefits as well, including lowering

LDL cholesterol, improving insulin sensitivity and having anti-arrhythmic effects. Adding more omega-3s without altering the total amount of daily fat may decrease coronary disease and total mortality among post MI patients.[12]

Sources of polyunsaturated fats are almonds, pecans, walnuts, fish, sunflower oil, safflower oil and soybean oil. Foods particularly high in omega-3s are almonds, walnuts, cold water fish (i.e. salmon, mackerel, herring), flax seeds and flax seed oil. If you use a device such as a George Foreman Grill™ to reduce excess fat in your meat, you may want to refrain from using it for fatty fish, such as salmon. This kind of fat is worth holding onto.

Supplementation of omega-3 fatty acids is usually not necessary, as long as you are consuming enough of the foods rich in this fat. If you choose to supplement with it, the usual recommended dose is 1000mg per 100 lbs. of bodyweight. Like vitamins and minerals, omega-3 fatty acid supplements are best taken with food. No more than 3 grams per day should be consumed without first discussing this with a healthcare provider. This is usually not an issue unless you are supplementing with additional omega-3 fatty acids.

Water

Although not recognized as a macronutrient, water is still important. As previously mentioned, 72% of our muscle is water. Adequate water intake is crucial for proper cellular functioning, among other numerous body processes.

The body is actually composed of 40-60% water. Without sufficient water intake, you will become dehydrated. Your body will retain water to protect itself. Retained water becomes contaminated because your kidneys cannot efficiently filter out contaminants when dehydrated. As a result, the liver works to process out these wastes, which interferes with one of its major functions – breaking down body fat. Additionally, when dehydrated, your body cannot adequately flush sodium from the body, leading to further water retention.

To prevent this, drink to minimize loss of body weight. For every pound of bodyweight lost with exercise, consider yourself having lost 16 ounces of water through sweat. If, for example, you had lost two pounds of weight during exercise, you will need an additional 32 ounces to replenish what fluid you had lost. I have found that drinking a half-ounce of water per pound of bodyweight per day is sufficient to ensure adequate hydration. Of course, those who sweat heavily may have greater requirements, depending on weight loss after their workout.

Keep in mind that as we age, the thirst mechanism in our brain declines.[1] As a result, we tend not to feel thirsty until we are dehydrated. A good rule of thumb is to check the color of your urine. If it is clear or very pale yellow, chances are good you are well-hydrated. If it is more of a distinct yellow or darker, it is safe to assume you can use additional water in your diet. As a professor in college once told me, "If you're peeing white, you're peeing right." What was meant by this was if your urine is fairly clear, you're doing well with hydration.

Vitamins

Vitamins fit under the category of micronutrients. They are organic substances needed in small amounts and are ingested without foods. They don't give us energy; rather, they act as helpers to trigger other reactions in the body.

There are two groups of vitamins: water soluble and fat soluble. Water soluble vitamins are the various B vitamins, vitamin C, biotin, and folate. These are not stored by the body, and excesses are excreted in the urine. Fat soluble vitamins (vitamins A, D, E and K), in contrast, are dissolved and stored in the fatty tissues of our body. As a result, too high an intake of fat soluble vitamins can lead to toxicity. It is beyond the scope of this book to go through each vitamin and discuss its purpose and recommended daily amount. There are great reference books that can provide such information. What is worth mentioning is that we tend not to get adequate intake from our daily food consumption. Thus, it is recommended to take at least a daily multivitamin. It is best taken with food for maximum absorption. There is no benefit to taking high doses of vitamins. With water soluble vitamins, what your body doesn't need will simply be excreted in the urine. At the very least, you will be left with expensive urine. With regard to fat soluble vitamins, too high an intake can lead to toxicity, which could be hazardous.

Minerals

Like vitamins, minerals are micronutrients. Minerals are inorganic substances needed for the body in fairly small amounts. There are 22 minerals in the body, making up about 4% of our body weight. They are found in soil and water, are taken up by the roots of plants and animals that eat these plants. As a result, we get our minerals from plants, animals and water. Examples of minerals are calcium, magnesium, potassium, zinc and iron. As I mentioned with vitamins, it is beyond the scope of this book to discuss the benefits and recommended daily intake for each mineral. What is worth mentioning is that like vitamins, too high or too low an intake can lead to health problems. Although we get many of our minerals in the diet, the fact that we are active and exercising regularly may justify the need for more. As an insurance policy, it may be wise to take a good multivitamin with minerals daily, with food.

Caffeine

Caffeine is a stimulant to the central nervous system found in coffee, tea, cocoa, and sodas (beverages of choice to many cultures). Although it doesn't fit under the category of a vitamin or mineral, it is important to mention this stimulant in relationship to heart disease. In addition to increasing one's heart rate and blood pressure, it has been shown to increase endurance and alertness, and to reduce fatigue. This can be extremely beneficial to those working long hours and attempting to accomplish a great number of tasks in a short period of time. It has also been added to a number of weight-loss supplements aimed at reducing body fat. It may help use fat for energy by sparing muscle glycogen, which is simply the carbohydrate stored in the muscle. As a result, more energy would be available for the muscles to perform. With that said, it's no wonder athletes have found coffee to be a cheap and effective performance enhancer. It explains why high doses of caffeine (the equivalent of eight cups of coffee) were banned by the International Olympic Committee (IOC) from 2000 until 2004. Although not currently banned, athletes are screened for high levels of caffeine and if the number of "abusers" is overwhelming, the current policy will be revisited.

Potential side effects of excess caffeine are sleep disorders, nausea, gastrointestinal instability, cramping, nervousness, anxiety, fatigue, dehydration, palpitations and arrhythmias. It is these last three that should be of particular concern to those with heart disease. Many of those with high blood pressure and/or heart disease take potent diuretics, which together with caffeine, which itself has diuretic properties, can further lead to dehydration. Palpitations can lead to dangerous arrhythmias, which could turn fatal. With an increase in heart rate and blood pressure, which are typical effects of caffeine, one could infer it has no place in the cardiac diet. Surprisingly enough, the research to this point does not support the notion that caffeine increases the risk of coronary heart disease.[13,14]

Although blood pressure runs higher for at least three hours after caffeine consumption, the rise is modest with an average of 8mmHg for systolic blood pressure and 6mmHg for diastolic blood pressure.[15] In several studies, after two weeks of regular consumption, no differences in blood pressure were found between consumers and non-consumers.[16,17,18] This supports the likelihood that a tolerance to caffeine is achieved over time.

It appears decaffeinated beverages serve no advantage over caffeinated beverages in terms of risk for coronary heart disease. In one particular study of over 45,000 men ages 40 to 75, the use of caffeine did not increase the risk of cardiovascular disease or stroke. However, a higher consumption of decaffeinated coffee was associated with a slightly elevated risk for coronary heart disease, compared with regular coffee.[19]

To provide a reference to how much caffeine is in these various beverages, a 6-oz. cup of instant coffee is equivalent to 60mg of caffeine, compared with 180mg per cup of brewed coffee, while 12 oz. of soda can range from 17 to 55mg. Newer energy drinks contain more. Caffeine or guarana (an herbal form of caffeine) can be one of numerous ingredients listed in a "proprietary blend," which may not list how many milligrams of caffeine are present – only the total of all listed ingredients.

In my experience, any negative heart-related effects occurred in those consuming these high-energy drinks and weight-loss pills. I've seen an experienced exerciser in his late 30s rushed to the hospital with a resting heart rate in the 180's shortly after consumption of a related product. He was given IV medication to break out of the arrhythmia. Perhaps the consumer was not accustomed to taking so much caffeine all at once. It is because of instances like this one that I do not support the use of these energy drinks and weight-loss products in those with or at risk for heart disease. The risks far outweigh any potential benefits. For those who simply want to enjoy a caffeinated beverage in moderate amounts (i.e. one to four cups), the suspected dangers do not appear to be validated. Moderation is key, especially for those with high blood pressure, high cholesterol, diabetes, and other high-risk individuals.

Finding a Proper Diet

The word "diet" tends to be grouped in the category of words with a negative connotation. When someone says he or she is dieting, it is usually said with an unpleasant tone. This is unfortunate because dieting can bring with it many health benefits and provide us with energy, and is the pathway along with exercise to achieving optimal health.

Webster's Dictionary defines diet as "food and drink consumed in a habitual manner." This doesn't have to be unpleasant at all. By consuming the right foods and drinks in the right quantities, we can enhance the quality and even the length of our lives.

This section will discuss the methods used to achieve the diet and weight goals you set for yourself, whether it is to gain weight, lose weight, or simply maintain your body weight with optimum energy.

Calories

For starters, let's discuss calories. A calorie is a unit of energy contained in any given amount of food. It is a measurement of heat. All of the macronutrients we discussed in the previous section – protein, carbohydrates, and fat – contain calories. Protein and carbohydrates each contain four calories per gram. Fat is the most caloric-dense, yielding nine calories per gram.

Our bodies burn calories in two different ways: our basal (resting) metabolism and physical activity.

Basal metabolism is simply the energy required to maintain basic life functions. In other words, it's the amount of calories needed at rest for your body to function properly. It does not include energy required or used to perform any type of movement or physical activity.

Your resting metabolic rate (RMR) is calculated based on your lean body mass. The more muscle mass you have, the faster your metabolic rate, thus the more calories your body needs for optimum functioning.

It should come as no surprise that a male bodybuilder would need to consume more calories than a frail, elderly woman. Other factors besides muscle mass that influence RMR are: age, gender, body type and thyroid function. The older we get, the slower our metabolism becomes. One explanation is that we experience muscle loss as we age. Women tend to have a slower metabolism due to lower muscle mass related to lower testosterone levels. More muscular individuals have faster metabolisms than their counterparts. Those with slower functioning thyroid glands would have less thyroid hormone production, thus a slower metabolic rate.

As mentioned earlier, physical activity also burns calories. For example, sleeping can burn roughly 72 calories per hour. By contrast, walking at 3.5 miles per hour can burn 336-420 calories per hour. Running at 7.5 miles per hour can burn as much as 900 calories per hour. This becomes important depending on whether you want to lose, gain or maintain bodyweight. You should have an idea of how many calories your body needs at rest (RMR) and how many calories are needed to perform physical activity demands. Simply put, to gain weight, you need to consume more calories than you burn. Conversely, if you want to lose weight, you need to burn more than you consume. For those who wish to maintain bodyweight, the calories consumed should closely match the calories burned.

For those wishing to get technical, you can calculate your RMR by the following Harris-Benedict Equation.[20,21]

RMR (males) = [13.75*weight (kg)] + [5*height (cm)] − [6.76*age] + 66

RMR (females) = [9.56*weight (kg)] + [1.85*height (cm)] − [4.68*age] + 655

To find your bodyweight in kilograms (kg), divide your weight in pounds by 2.2. For example, if you weigh 200 pounds, you will divide 200 by 2.2, resulting in 90.9 or simply 91 kg. To measure your height in centimeters (cm), multiply your height in inches by 2.54. For example, if you measure 5'7" (67 inches), you will multiply this by 2.54, resulting in 170.18 cm. If this same person was a 50-year-old male, we can easily calculate his RMR:

RMR = [13.75*91 kg] + [5*170.18 cm] − [6.76*50] + 66
RMR = [1251.25] + [850.9] − [338] + 66
RMR = 1330.15 calories

This means that at complete rest, this individual requires approximately 1330 calories just to maintain proper life functioning. Keep in mind that this does not factor in calories that are needed to perform daily physical activities.

With all of the fad diets out there claiming miraculous and quick weight loss, high energy and optimum health, the only results achieved tend to be those of confusion and disappointment. One of the many reasons for such failure is due to the restrictiveness of these diets. Take the Atkins Diet, for example, which promotes a maximum of 20 grams of carbohydrates per day for the first two weeks of the diet. You can eat all of the protein, fat, saturated fat you want, as long as the carbohydrates are kept very low.

Although weight loss can and usually is achieved, this tends to be an unrealistic way for eating long term. Since a vast majority of vitamins, minerals and fiber come from carbohydrates, we tend to become deficient without proper daily supplementation. Research shows that although weight loss is more significant at six months with a low carbohydrate diet compared with a low fat diet, no significant difference occurs at one year.[22] Weight loss was associated with the duration of the diet and the degree of calorie restriction, not on the reduced carbohydrate content.[23]

Weight control is based on energy balance, not macronutrient composition of the diet. One pound of fat is equivalent to 3500 calories. For weight loss to occur, we need to burn more calories than we consume. To ensure that the weight we lose is body fat and not muscle tissue, it is recommended that we lose no more than two pounds of weight per week. Initially, you may drop more than this when starting a diet. But this is mainly water loss, which usually occurs due to lower calorie consumption. But overall, the weekly weight loss should not be too drastic.

For healthy weight loss to occur, it may be a wise investment to purchase a calorie counter, which is simply a reference book providing nutritional information on various foods.[24] It will reveal the serving size and calories as well as grams of fat, saturated fat, protein, carbohydrates, fiber and cholesterol for most foods. You can then determine how many calories you are currently consuming by measuring your food and calculating the calories. You can even be more thorough and include the percentage of calories coming from carbohydrates, protein and fat. Remember that one gram of protein is four calories; one gram of carbohydrate is four calories; and one gram of fat is nine calories.

Successfully losing weight at the rate of one to two pounds a week can be accomplished by reducing your calories slightly, with a small increase in activity, thus adding to calories burned. For example, if you consume 250 fewer calories each day, and increase activity so that you burn an additional 250 calories per day, you will burn 500 calories per day. In a seven-day period, you will have burned 3500 calories. If you recall, 3500 calories is equivalent to one pound of fat.

As simple as it is to lose weight, gaining weight can be just as simple. The trick to gaining weight is to steadily increase your caloric intake. You could begin by increasing your caloric intake by 250 calories per day and monitor your weight in one to two weeks. If you're still not gaining, increase another 250 calories per day and reassess after another week. Repeat this pattern until you begin to see a weight gain. I wouldn't recommend decreasing physical activity much, unless you are overtraining (see Chapter 11).

The next issue we need to discuss is the ratio of carbohydrates, fats and proteins. Several diets exist which promote various ratios of our three macronutrients. You have "The Zone Diet," which teaches to aim for 40%

carbohydrates, 30% protein, and 30% fat. The Atkins Diet aims for less than 20 grams of carbohydrates, which could equate to less than 10% of your total calories for the day. The rest would be made up of protein and fat, with no specific ratio of each.

What we must always remember is that it is the calories consumed and burned that dictate whether we gain, lose or maintain weight. Where these calories come from isn't the greatest factor. However, let's not underestimate the importance of carbohydrates, protein and fat in the diet; as well as vitamins, minerals and fiber. We need carbohydrates in the body to provide us with vitamins, minerals and fiber. Without carbohydrates, we can survive, but will need to rely on vitamin, mineral and fiber supplements to ensure proper health. Another advantage to having carbohydrates in the diet is to provide our muscles with the necessary glycogen for optimum exercise performance. This is the carbohydrate stored in our muscles. The common ratio of carbohydrates seems to be between 30% and 65% of total caloric intake. Any higher than 65%, and you run the risk of depriving yourself of protein and fats, which are no less important.

As stated earlier, protein contains amino acids, which are the building blocks of our body's tissues. Although the recommended dietary intake is 0.8 grams per kilogram of bodyweight per day, the fact that we are exercising regularly gives us the need for additional protein in the diet. I've seen great results in my clients who consumed closer to one gram of protein per pound of bodyweight each day. The results include faster recovery from workouts, decreased muscle soreness, increased muscle mass and decreased body fat. Studies have shown that when exercise is incorporated with a high-protein diet, greater body fat loss along with a greater maintenance of muscle mass is achieved.[25,26] A diet consisting of 25-40% protein should suffice. Since meat and egg yolks carry a significant amount of fat, it would be wise to aim for lean meats, and to consume more egg whites than yolk. Egg substitutes, such as "egg beaters," are another option.

Years ago, I used to think dietary fat was the enemy. I was under the impression that if you eat fat, you will become fat. While it is true that the most common diets are low in fats, it is not for the reason I once believed. It is simply because fat is the most caloric-dense of the macronutrients, yielding nine calories per gram. Since losing weight requires that we burn more calories than we consume, by following a diet high in fat, it wouldn't take much to exceed our limit.

Most experts would argue it doesn't matter what the ratio of macronutrients is as long as we consume the necessary amount of calories to achieve our desired goal. But in reality, it does matter, because is if we don't have enough carbohydrates in our diet, we won't have enough vitamins, minerals and fiber for optimal health. If we don't have enough protein in our diet, we won't have the necessary amino acids for muscle recovery and growth. That leaves us with only so much room for dietary fat. At nine calories per gram, it doesn't take much to meet our requirements. A diet consisting of 20-30% fat should be sufficient. No more than 8% should be from saturated fat. The goal is to keep the saturated fat as low as possible, relying mostly on the monounsaturated and polyunsaturated fatty acids.

It may seem overwhelming to eat so much food, especially protein. What seems to work best for people is dividing up your intake into four to six smaller meals. A good rule of thumb is to eat a small meal every two to four waking hours. By dividing up your protein into this many meals, it is easily achievable. Furthermore, it will provide you with long-lasting energy and it will also help speed up your metabolism. The term *grazing* can be used to describe this eating pattern. This is how people with diabetes are generally taught to eat, to help control their blood sugar. This holds true for athletes, as well as those looking to gain, lose or even maintain weight.

There is no evidence that macronutrient composition enhances fat loss. It is the calories that need adjustment. Gradual weight loss increases your success for keeping the weight off permanently. Therefore, aim to lose no more than two pounds of weight per week. Eating a variety of foods is recommended for optimum health. Focus on nutrient-dense foods. These are low calorie foods with high nutrients, such as broccoli. Although it is low in calories at 25 calories per cup, it contains significant amounts of calcium, vitamin C and potassium.

Limiting juices and sodas for zero-calorie beverages is another method to reduce excess calories in your diet. Just like broccoli, an orange will have more potassium, vitamin C and fiber, as opposed to the high-calorie 8-oz. glass of orange juice. You'd be surprised at how small dietary changes combined with increased exercise can transform your physique to the way you want to look and feel.

Important note: *Although certain fruits and fruit juices are packed with nutrients to provide optimal health, certain ones should be avoided when taking certain heart medications because they can increase the potency to potentially dangerous levels. Check with your doctor or pharmacist to determine if you need to avoid the following:*

- *grapefruit or grapefruit juice*

- *pomegranate or pomegranate juice*
- *Seville oranges*

Developing a meal plan

Now that you know how many calories you need to accomplish your weight goals, you need to develop a good meal plan. What has worked for me is eating frequent small meals, consisting of some lean protein, a high-fiber carbohydrate (e.g. rice, oatmeal, potato), which would be some sort of slow-burning starch that provides long-lasting energy, and a non-starchy vegetable. I make sure I get fiber in the majority of my meals. This not only provides you with a feeling of fullness, but helps to stabilize blood sugar; especially important for those with diabetes.

Although we get a decent amount of fat in the meat we eat, this is usually in the form of the unhealthy saturated fat. We've already discussed the benefits of monounsaturated and polyunsaturated fats. To meet these needs, having one to two tablespoons of extra virgin olive oil in a salad or a couple of tablespoons of flax seed oil in a protein shake might be a good idea.

At this point, you should have a much better understanding of diet and nutrition. You now have the tools to put a good diet together to reach whatever goals you set for yourself. When constructing your diet, you need to determine how many calories you should be consuming daily. Remember that to lose weight, you should burn more calories than you consume. To gain weight, you should consume more calories than you burn. To maintain your body weight, continue to consume the same amount of calories you currently take in.

The next priority is ensuring that you have an adequate amount of carbohydrates, protein and fat in your diet. The ratio I tend to favor is a 40:30:30 ratio, where 40% to 50% of my calories are carbohydrates, 25-30% are protein, with 20-30% being fat calories. Saturated fat should be less than 10% of your total caloric intake. You will find specific amounts of each macronutrient on the nutrition label listed on most food products.

The following conversion table can help you figure out how many calories are in each gram of macronutrient:

- 1 gram of carbohydrate = 4 calories
- 1 gram of protein = 4 calories
- 1 gram of fat = 9 calories

In the Appendix in the back of this book, you will find sample diets to use as a reference. Keep in mind that these are only samples and not meant to be followed exactly as written. Refer to a nutritionist or registered dietitian for a specific diet tailored to your personal needs. The samples are meant to show you an example of a weight loss diet for a 140 pound female and a weight maintenance diet for a 175 pound male. All of the information regarding grams of protein, carbohydrates, fats, and numbers of calories were all obtained either from the nutrition label or from my calorie-counter book.[24]

Here are 10 tips based on my training as a registered nurse and exercise physiologist, research, as well as my own efforts over the years, for helping you with your dieting goals:

10 Tips for Dieting Success:

1. Measure your food. Invest in a food scale, as well as measuring cups and spoons to enable you to have better portion control.
2. Eat protein first at every meal. This will help stabilize your blood sugar and get you full faster so you won't be so tempted to overdo it on carbohydrates and fats. It will also ensure adequate amino acids for muscle repair, recovery, and growth.
3. Stick with fresh or frozen vegetables. Canned vegetables contain added sugar, sodium and other preservatives, which can promote water retention and stimulate salt/sugar cravings. If you have to use canned vegetables, consider choosing the ones that are marked "lower sodium."
4. Aim for four to six small meals per day. Small and frequent meals help stabilize your blood sugar, prevent overeating, and keep your metabolism elevated.
5. Increase fiber and lower simple sugars. Diets high in fiber help stabilize your blood sugar as well as lower cholesterol, and provide you with a feeling of satiety or fullness so you'll be less likely to binge on too much of the wrong foods, such as high-sugar sweets. Replace fruit juice with whole fresh fruit.
6. Limit starches when you are less active. You don't really need these "energy foods" when your body is preparing for an overnight sleep. A better choice would be a lean protein source with greens and a healthy fat.

7. <u>Limit processed foods</u>. As the late Jack LaLanne, who lived to 97, once said when asked about the secret to such great health and fitness in his nineties, "I don't eat anything that wasn't harvested or killed." In other words, he avoided man-made foods and opted for what the earth provides in its most natural form.

8. <u>Aim for at least ½ oz. of water per pound of bodyweight daily (unless contraindicated).</u> This amounts to between eight and 14 8-oz. glasses of water a day for the average person. Adequate hydration helps promote feelings of satiety so you're less likely to overeat. Being zero calories makes it the beverage of choice. (However, disregard this tip if you have been placed on fluid restrictions by your doctor due to congestive heart failure, kidney disease or other conditions).

9. <u>Weigh yourself often, even daily</u>. It was long advised by nutritionists and health gurus alike to avoid being too fixated with the number on the scale. It was believed the dieter would quickly become discouraged. Therefore, the advice was to weigh yourself weekly, not daily. But new research indicates that those who weigh themselves daily are more likely to make the appropriate caloric adjustments, and to exercise, to get on track.[27] Think of it this way: a diabetic checks his or her blood sugar often in order to make the appropriate medication/dietary adjustments. Why shouldn't you do the same with your body weight?

10. <u>If you "cheat," do so infrequently</u>. We are all likely to face food temptations from time to time. We can always successfully fight these when necessary, but if we were to indulge in a piece of birthday cake or too many sweets over the holidays, it is not the end of the world. Resume your diet and know that you don't have to surrender in defeat. Months of work do not go wasted by a single "cheat meal."

Chapter 14

Conclusion/Going Forward

We have arrived at the last chapter in this book, a book that I hope has opened your eyes to the benefits of exercise, specific exercises that you can do on your own, or as part of a cardiac rehab program, or working with a personal trainer or a cardiac rehab nurse/trainer. It has also provided you with information about how to reduce your stress and to improve your diet and nutrition so that, together with your exercise regimen, you will have the best chance at optimum health now and going forward, whatever your age.

I want to share with you the story in his own words of one of my cardiac rehab patients whom I'll call George. He is now a 77-year-old grandfather who had open-heart surgery 10 years ago. George is 6'1" tall and he weighs about 190 pounds. He would never describe himself as a "couch potato" for he prides himself on staying physically active. His risk factors for heart disease include family history, type II diabetes, and smoking for 45 years. Here is George's story:

It was early January of 2000 when I went for my annual physical. My primary care physician noticed that my EKG did not compare favorably with the previous one and suggested I see a cardiologist. Upon seeing one, a stress test and radioactive test were performed and indicated that further testing was necessary. On Monday, January 7th, I had a cardiac catheterization done to explore the vessels. I figured while in there, the cardiologist would put a few stents in me (from the limited cardiac knowledge I had) to clean up whatever blockages I might have and then I'd be on my way. Upon wakening from anesthesia, I asked, "Am I good to go?" The cardiologist shook his head from side-to-side. At that time, I knew the next step would be open-heart surgery. Apparently, there was too much damage – 85%, 90%, and 100% blockages. On Thursday, January 10th, my wife and I met with the surgeon who suggested that although not an emergency, I should have it done soon. I told them I was ready. My thinking was to get it done before I had a major heart attack. I was told it couldn't be done until Tuesday, January 15th. I immediately gave my consent.

On that Tuesday morning, I pulled in to the hospital parking garage at 6:15 am and enjoyed my last cigarette. Why did I decide to stop at that time? When speaking with my surgeon the previous week, I asked him how long the bypass would last. He said 15-25 years, unless I continued to smoke. If I continued, it would only last five to seven years. I filed that in my memory bank as a "no-brainer" decision.

So a triple bypass was done and I remained in the hospital for one week. Because of numerous years of heavy smoking, I had a little trouble coming off of the ventilator, but otherwise, my stay was relatively uneventful. Probably the hardest part for me in the hospital was getting out of bed to walk. I remember a young lady from physical therapy came to my room a few days after surgery and said we were going to do some walking. The only walking I had done prior to that was from my bed to the bathroom. She provided a walker for my balance, which was poor initially. We stepped out of the room into the hallway and walked to the end and back. In reality, the hallway was not very long, but at the time, it seemed an insurmountable distance. Slowly and deliberately, I made it up and back and was completely exhausted. A day or so later, we tackled stairs. Because I lived in a raised ranch, she said I had to practice going up and down stairs. This proved to be much more difficult than walking.

My wife remained with me during my entire stay at the hospital. She was able to take care of all of my non-medical needs for which I was extremely grateful, as were the hospital personnel. As should be, they were able to devote their time to my medical concerns, as well as their other patients.

When my wife brought me home from the hospital, it took me a great amount of time to walk up the slight incline to my front door. I had to stop a number of times climbing up the five stairs into our home. To add excitement to the recovery, we were having an addition constructed to our house which began December 15th. All of the furniture from the end of the house where the addition was taking place was moved to the other end. For example, the bed was in the dining room while most of the bedroom furniture was in the living room. This was actually good for me as there were pathways between furniture which helped support me for I was extremely weak.

Although the two carpenters working on the addition had been told I was going to the hospital for an operation, they obviously didn't realize the severity of the procedure. When I first got out of the car, they yelled down, "What did they do to you?" as I walked very slowly and gingerly. Looking *back, a week before the operation, I was on my roof removing old gutters and helping the two men lift a 25-foot petition wall into place. In retrospect, I'm very lucky I didn't have a heart attack while on the roof. If the blockages didn't kill me, the fall would have!*

The carpenters asked me what I was going to do now that I was home. I said I would probably read and watch a little television on the small set in the kitchen, as it would take me too long to go down the stairs where the large television was located. Unknown to me at the time, they checked with my wife and then ran a new cable upstairs into the living room and moved the large television up so I could watch the large set comfortably. This was not requested by me and showed a great deal of caring of the two men whose sole purpose was to build an addition to my house.

The next couple of months recovering at home were a difficult time period. I didn't want any phone calls or visitors, including my family. This was very unusual as I was normally a very outgoing person. I guess because of my weakened state and lack of energy, I did not want people seeing me in that condition. There were a few that snuck by, such as my minister and a few close friends, but very few.

It was two months before I could lift a gallon of milk and then it was necessary to use both hands. For someone who used to lift two gallons with a finger and thumb on one hand, some difficult mental adjustments were necessary. Had my wife not put milk for my coffee in a small container, I would not have had any.

For a few months, I was unable to drive and was told not to ride in the front passenger seat because of the airbag. My wife had a large luxury automobile at the time. She would be driving while I would be sitting in the back seat hugging a teddy bear to help splint my chest incision area. This created quite a picture when we ran into people we knew. I did not drive until about two months after surgery. I was surprised how hesitant I was to get behind the wheel, considering I'd been driving since age sixteen!

In early February, I began the cardiac rehab program at my hospital, as recommended by my cardiologist. Prior to my surgery, I was a relatively active person. I kept busy doing yard work, tree work, automotive work, and maintenance work for my church. For several months after surgery, I was extremely weak. This was particularly evident when the nurses got me on the treadmill and I asked if I could slow down. Their response was, "It doesn't go any slower." I knew I'd have a long battle to get back to "normal."

With time, I did start to see steady progress. The education segments which my wife and I attended were very informative and gave her a feeling of confidence in my future and the things necessary to lead a healthy life. The nutrition classes were very beneficial, as well. My eating concerns were modified slightly but being diabetic, I was already highly regulated on my diet. Both my wife and I had been eating in a healthy manner, which became more of a factor after the surgery.

One of the defining moments for me in my recovery period was after about nine weeks in cardiac rehab when I finally felt strong enough to throw a baseball with my eleven-year-old grandson and build a sand castle with my three-year-old granddaughter. Now, my oldest grandson is 21 and is a three-hour drive away from me. My granddaughter is now 13 and I have a nine-year-old grandson, as well. I feel especially blessed that I'm able to stay physically active and be there for them. Even though I don't see too much of my 21-year-old grandson, I know that when football season is upon us, I can make the trip up to Massachusetts to met him for a New England Patriots game and know I can climb the bleachers without too much effort at 77 years of age.

Although it was nearly a year before I felt like my "old-self," had it not been for the excellent care I received at the hospital, the cardiac rehab center, my devoted wife, and the prayers of all, I probably wouldn't be here today. The people at rehab were so patient and understanding with me, it made a difficult time in my life much easier.

As a sort of "payback," I devote time to a cardiac support group at my hospital. Here, I am able to converse with those who've had any type of cardiac condition and ease their concerns. As a board member, I'd listen to concerns of the attendees, whether it be the number of medications they take, number of doctors they see, their fear of not living a long life, etc. Although no board member has a medical background, each has had some type of cardiac procedure – stents, pacemakers, defibrillators, open-heart surgery (some multiple times), etc. After explaining what we had gone through and the ages of many of our board members (oldest is 89), the people suddenly feel a lot better about their concerns knowing that they are not alone. Through various fundraisers the support group sponsors, more than $200,000 since 1981 was donated to the hospital to provide equipment as well as funds for further education of the staff. The time that I devote is a small price to pay for a wonderful continuation of life.

George is a wonderful example of how his open heart surgery at the age of 67 was a turning point for him. The positive changes he made in his life, including a commitment to regular exercise and to continue to avoid smoking, a 45-year habit he ended at 67, has enabled him to live 10 more healthy years filled with lots of happy, active times with his family including his children and grandchildren. Let's hope he'll be one of those centenarians who are becoming more and more numerous in the United States and around the world as living past 100 is no longer as unusual as it used to be.

If George is able to commit to a healthier lifestyle, why not you? Why shouldn't you start to do, right now, the actions that will help you to become a healthy centenarian? Exercise and diet, and reducing stress, are key ways to achieve that healthier you.

In summary, here are the key benefits of a regular exercise program to your heart and your health:

- A reduction in your resting heart rate and blood pressure
- Increased HDL (good) cholesterol and decreased LDL (bad) cholesterol
- Reduced total body fat
- Reduced blood platelet adhesiveness and aggregation (sticky blood)
- Improved glucose tolerance (decreased insulin requirements)
- Decreasing the workload on your heart
- Increased bone density (stronger bones)
- Decreased anxiety
- Less depression
- Lower stress levels
- Enhanced feelings of well-being
- A better ability to perform work, recreational and sports activities

As noted in the Introduction to this book, in the United States alone, almost one million people will have a heart attack this year and another 300,000 will suffer cardiac arrest where the heart stops beating.[1,2] For that reason, you should consider getting yourself trained in cardiopulmonary resuscitation (CPR). That skill may help you to save a life.

If an adult goes into sudden cardiac arrest, his or her survival is dependent upon early and effective CPR. Unfortunately, only about one-third of those individuals who suffer cardiac arrest outside of the hospital receive CPR from a bystander. Many bystanders naturally feel uncomfortable taking that responsibility. They may be afraid something will go wrong or they'll make the situation worse. Traditional CPR has involved chest compressions and mouth-to-mouth respirations. Many bystanders feared the passage of germs from these respirations. But the most recent CPR guidelines are known as "hands-only CPR," chest compressions only.[3] This method can be equally as effective as conventional CPR in the first few minutes after an out-of -hospital cardiac event.[4] And you no longer need fear giving mouth-to-mouth resuscitation.

The word is finally spreading to communities throughout the United States and around the world of the importance of CPR. Organizations such as Hands for Life‟ in the United States have been formed with the goal of training mass numbers of people in a given day. Singapore currently holds the Guinness Book of World Records with 7,909 participants, organized by the Singapore Heart Foundation in January 2011. I was privileged to be a part of the Hands for Life‟ event on August 25‟ 2012, in Stamford, Connecticut, where over 5,100 participants were trained in 10 hours, breaking the record in the United States. It was so inspirational to see the interest in Connecticut, with participants ranging in age from five years old up to over 80! When an elderly female was asked why she wanted to be trained when she clearly could not kneel down for chest compressions, nor did she have the strength to perform the life-saving task, her response was, "I may not have the strength to do it myself, but I can sure instruct people on what to do and make sure they are doing it right."

Her comment sends a powerful message to us all that everyone has the ability to make a difference, even if they have physical limitations, to work toward eliminating heart disease as our number one killer, with many preventable risk factors such as lack of exercise and obesity.

I leave you now with the tools in this book to put together a productive training program for yourself, focusing on strength, endurance, and flexibility. In addition, after reading *Pump it Up!* you now have the tools to set up a good nutritional program for yourself, whether your goal is to lose, gain, or maintain your healthy body weight. You are now aware of the importance in practicing techniques for stress reduction. Just like exercise and diet require consistency, we need to be consistent in our measures to reduce the stress in our lives. You also now have a better understanding of *good pain* and *bad pain*, and when an intervention is required.

Most important of all, I want to emphasize that exercise needs to be a daily obligation. If you think about animals in the wild, those creatures never miss a day of exercise. Take a domesticated dog and lock him up for a week. You will watch him quickly going stir crazy!

Eugene Sandow, a famous bodybuilder of the Victorian era, was known in his time as being the world's strongest man and the "Father of Modern

Bodybuilding." Since 1977, a trophy of Sandow is presented to the overall winner of the Mr. Olympia contest, which is the most extravagant title a professional bodybuilder can win. Sandow was once quoted as saying, "Life is movement." Choose life and keep moving!

Finally, by following the heart healthy principles that you have learned or had reinforced in this book, the life you save could be a family member's or your own.

Notes

Introduction

[1] L.A. Kaminsky, K.A. Bonheim, C.E. Garber, S.C. Glass, L.F. Hamm, H.W. Kohl III, & A. Mikesky. (Eds.). *ACSM's Resource Manual for Guidelines for Exercise Testing and Prescription* (4th Ed.). Baltimore: Lippincott Williams & Wilkins, 2006.

[2] J.S. Schiller, J.W. Lucas, B.W. Ward, & J.A. Peregoy. "Summary Health Statistics for U.S. Adults: National Health Interview Survey, 2010. National Center for Health Statistics." *Vital Health Statistics.* 10(252) (2012): 19.

[3] L. Robertson, A. Rogers, A. Ewing, et al. (Eds.). *American Association of Cardiovascular and Pulmonary Rehabilitation and Secondary Prevention Programs* (4th ed.). Champaign, IL: Human Kinetics, 2004.

[4] American Heart Association. "Doctors Should Encourage Cardiac Rehab Programs." 2005. <http://newsroom.heart.org/news/doctors-should-encourage-cardiac-223005> Accessed March 6, 2006.

[5] K.R. Vincent, R.W. Braith, R.A. Feldman, P.M. Magyari, R.B. Cutler, S.A. Persin, et al. "Resistance Exercise and Physical Performance in Adults Aged 60 to 83." *Journal of the American Geriatrics Society.* 50(6) (2002): 1100-1107.

Chapter 1

[1] A.S. Go, D. Mozaffarian, V.L Roger, E.J. Benjamin, J.D. Berry, et. al. AHA Statistical Update. "Heart Disease and Stroke Statistics – 2013 Update." Circulation. 2013. <http://circ.ahajournals.org/content/127/1/e6.full> Accessed January 7, 2013. doi: 10.1161/CIR.obo13e31828124ad.

[2] Centers for Disease Control and Prevention (CDC). "Prevalence and Most Common Causes of Disability Among Adults – United States, 2005." Morbidity and Mortality Weekly Report. 58 (2009): 421-426.

[3] "Financial Preparedness Critical to Heart Disease Sufferers." Council For Disability Awareness. June 2008. <http://www.disabilitycanhappen.org/chances_disability/causes.asp> (12 August 2012).

[4] W. Hurst. *The Heart, Arteries, and Veins* (10th ed.). New York, NY: McGraw-Hill, 2002.

Chapter 3

[1] J.H. Wilmore, & D.C. Costill. *Physiology of Sport and Exercise* (2nd ed.). Champaign, IL: Human Kinetics, 1999.

[2] American College of Sports Medicine. *ACSM's Exercise Management for Persons with Chronic Diseases and Disabilities*. Champaign, IL: Human Kinetics, 1997.

[3] R.O. Cummins, (Ed.). *ACLS Provider Manual*. Dallas, TX: American Heart Association. (2001).

[4] J.L. Cox, N. Ad, T. Palazzo, S. Fitzpatrick, J.P Suyderhoud, K.W. DeGroot, et al. "Current Status of the Maze Procedure for the Treatment of Atrial Fibrillation." Seminars of Thoracic and Cardiovascular Surgery. 12(1) (2000): 15-19.

[5] D.C. Nieman. *Exercise Testing and Prescription: A Health-Related Approach* (4th ed.). Mountain View, CA: Mayfield Publishing Company, 1999.

[6] M.H. Whaley, P.H. Brubaker, & R.M. Otto. (Eds.). *ACSM's Guidelines for Exercise Testing and Prescription* (7th ed.). Baltimore: Lippincott Williams & Wilkins, 2006.

[7] S.M. Lewis, M.M. Heitkemper, & S.R. Dirksen. *Medical-Surgical Nursing: Assessment and Management of Clinical Problems* (6th ed.). St. Louis, MI: Mosby, Inc., 2004.

Chapter 4

[1] V.L. Roger, A.S. Go, D.M. Lloyd-Jones, R.J. Adams, J.D. Berry. "Heart Disease and Stroke Statistics – 2011 Update: A Report From the American Heart Association." *Circulation.* 123 (2010): e18-e209.

[2] M.H. Whaley, et. al.

[3] "ACSM's Exercise Management for Persons with Chronic Diseases and Disabilities"

[4] R. Gabriel, M. Alonso, B. Reviriego, J. Muñiz, S. Vega, et.al. "Ten-Year Fatal and Non-Fatal Myocardial Infarction Incidence in Elderly Populations in Spain: The Epicardian Cohort Study." *Biomed Central Public Health.* 9 (2009): 360.

[5] Mosby's Nursing Drug Reference. St.Louis, MI: Mosby, Inc., 2004.

[6] "The Surgeon General's Call to Action to Prevent and Decrease Overweight and Obesity."(2007). <http://www.surgeongeneral.gov/topics/obesity/calltoaction/fact_adolescents.htm> (2 October 2008).

[7] N.A. Melville. "Sedentary Behavior Associated with Higher Mortality." 2011. American College of Sports Medicine (ACSM) 58th Annual Meeting. Abstract 623. Presented June 2, 2011.

[8] C. Wade & C. Tavris. *Invitation to Psychology.* 3rd Edition. New Jersey: Pearson Prentice Hall, 2005.

[9] K.W. Davidson, et. al. "Assessment and Treatment of Depression in Patients With Cardiovascular Disease: National Heart, Lung, and Blood Institute Working Group Report." *Psychosomatic Medicine.* 68(5) (2006): 645-650.

[10] National Institute of Mental Health. "Depression and Heart Disease, Bethesda (MD)": National Institute of Mental Health, National Institutes of Health, US Department of Health and Human Services. 2002. (NIH Publication No. 02-5004) 4 pages. <http://www.nimh.nih.gov> (2 November 2006).

[11] L.A. Kaminsky, et. al.

[12] B. Naparstek. *Staying Well with Guided Imagery.* New York: Warner Books, 1994.

[13] J. Strauss. "Research Findings on Imagery & PTSD." Preliminary findings presented at the Army's 10th Annual Force Health Protection Conference. Louisville, KY, (August 2007).

[14] J.J. Daubenmier, G. Weidner, M. Sumner, N. Mendell, T. Merritt-Worden, J. Studley, et al. "The Contribution of Changes in Diet, Exercise, and StressManagement to Changes in Coronary Risk in Women and Men in the Multisite Cardiac Lifestyle Intervention Program." *Annals of Behavioral Medicine.* 33(1) (2007): 57-68.

Chapter 5
[1] M.H Whaley, et. al.

[2] L.A. Kaminsky, et. al.

[3] J. Munn, R.D. Herbert, & S.C. Gandevia. "Contralateral Effects of Unilateral Resistance Training: A Meta-Analysis." *Journal of Applied Physiology.* 96 (2004): 1861-1866.

[4] R.K. Oka, A.C. King, & D.R. Young. "Sources of Social Support as Predictors of Exercise Adherence in Women and Men Ages 50 to 65 Years." *Women's Health.* 1(2) (1995): 161-175.

Chapter 6
[1] J. Smorawinski, K. Nazar, H. Kaciuba-Uscilko, E. Kaminska, G. Cybulski, A. Kodrzycka, et. al. "Effects of 3-Day Bed Rest on Physiological Responses to Graded Exercise in Athletes and Sedentary Men." *Journal of Applied Physiology.* 91(1) (2001): 249-257.

[2] M.H. Whaley, et. al.

[3] L.A. Kaminsky, et. al.

[4] R.L. Gellish, B.R. Goslin, R.E. Olson, A. McDonald, G.D. Russi, & V.K. Moudgil, "Longitudinal Modeling of the Relationship Between Age and Maximal Heart Rate." *Medicine and Science in Sports and Exercise.* 39(5) (2007): 822-829.

[5] T.R. Baechle & R. Earle (Eds.). *Essentials of Strength Training and Conditioning* (2nd ed.). Champaign, IL: Human Kinetics, 2000.

[6] A. Hauser. "30 Minutes of Exercise Does the Trick, Study Says." Everyday Health. 2012. <http://www.everydayhealth.com/fitness/0824/30-minutes-of-exercise-does-the-trick-study-says.aspx?xid=aol_eh-genvid_5_20120827_&aolcat=HLT&icid=maing-grid10%7Chtmlws-main-bb%7Cdl36%7Csec1_lnk3%26pLid%3D197614> (28 August 2012).

[7] W.L. Haskell, I. Lee, R.R. Pate, K.E. Powell, S.N. Blair, B.A. Franklin, et. al. "Physical Activity and Public Health: Updated Recommendation for Adults from The American College of Sports Medicine and the American Heart Association." *Medicine and Science in Sports and Exercise.* 39(8) (2007): 1423-1434.

[8] T.J. Quinn, J.R. Klooster, & B.C. Focht. "Two Short, Daily Activity Bouts Vs. One Long Bout: Are Health and Fitness Improvements Similar Over Twelve and Twenty-four Weeks?" *Journal of Strength and Conditioning Research.* 20(1) (2006): 130-135.

Chapter 7
[1] A. Soni. "Back Problems: Use and Expenditures for the U.S. Adult Population, 2007. Statistical Brief #289." July 2010. Agency for Healthcare Research and Quality.
<http://www.meps.ahrq.gov/mepsweb/data_files/publications/st289/stat289.pdf> (15 August 2012)

Chapter 10
[1] "ACSM's Exercise Management for Persons with Chronic Diseases and Disabilities."

Chapter 11
[1] J.H. Wilmore, et. al.

[2] "ACSM's Exercise Management for Persons with Chronic Diseases and Disabilities."

[3] P. Girlanda, R. Dattola, C. Venuto, R. Mangiapane, C. Nicolosi, & C. Messina, "Local Steroid Treatment in Idiopathic Carpal Tunnel Syndrome: Short- and Long-Term Efficacy." *Journal of Neurology.* 240(3) (1993): 187-190.

[4] S. Stahl, & T. Kaufman. "The Efficacy of an Injection of Steroids for Medial Epicondylitis: A Prospective Study of Sixty Elbows." *The Journal of Bone and Joint Surgery.* 79 (1997): 1648-1652.

[5] "A Promising Treatment for Athletes, in Blood." 2009. <http://www.nytimes.com/2009/02/17/sports/17blood.html?pagewanted=all&_r=0 > (13 July 2011).

[6] "You Might Have Exercise Fever, but Is It OK to Workout When Ill?" 2008. <http://www.gadsdentimes.com/article/20080131/news/801310306/1049/lifetimes.> (6 February 2008).

[7] Mosby's *Nursing Drug Reference.*

[8] M.H. Whaley, et. al.

Chapter 12
[1] "Mosby's *Nursing Drug Reference.*"

[2] D.N. Juurlink, J.V. Tu, & M.M. Mamdani. "Interactions Between Clopidogrel and Proton Pump Inhibitors." *Canadian Medical Association Journal.* 180(12) (2009): 1229.

[3] P.H. Stone, N.A. Gratsiansky, A. Blokhin, et al. "Antianginal Efficacy of Ranolazine when Added to Maximal Therapy with Conventional Therapy: The Efficacy of Ranolazine in Chronic Angina Trial." *Circulation.* 48 (2006): 566-575.

[4] E.S. Nissen, & K. Wolski. "Effect of Rosiglitazone on the Risk of Myocardial Infarction and Death from Cardiovascular Causes." *New England Journal of Medicine.* 356(24) (2007): 2457-2471.

[5] R.R. Wolfe. "Protein Supplements and Exercise." *American Journal of Clinical Nutrition.* 72(supp) (2000): 551s-7s.

[6] L.S. Kripalani, L.C. Roumie, K.A. Dalal, C. Cawthon, A. Businger, et. al. "Effect of a Pharmacist Intervention on Clinically Important Medication Errors After Hospital Discharge: A Randomized Trial." *Annals of Internal Medicine.* 157(1) (2012): 1-10.

Chapter 13
[1] J.H. Wilmore, et. al.

[2] R.R. Wolfe. "Protein Supplements and Exercise." *American Journal of Clinical Nutrition.* 72(supp) (2000): 551s-7s.

[3] R.P. Heaney. "Protein and Calcium: Antagonists or Synergists?" *The American Journal of Clinical Nutrition.* 75(4) (2002): 609-610.

[4] C.W. Wong, & D.L. Watson. "Immunomodulatory Effects of Dietary Whey Proteins in Mice." *Journal of Dairy Research.* 62 (1995): 359-368.

[5] P.P.L. Low, K.J. Rutherford, H.S. Gill, & M.L. Cross. "Effects of Dietary Whey Protein Concentrate on Primary and Secondary Antibody Responses in Immunized BALB/c Mice." *International Immunopharmacology.* 3 (2003): 393-401.

[6] L.R. Bucci & L. Unlu. "Protein and Amino Acids in Exercise and Sport." In: "Energy-Yielding Macronutrients and Energy Metabolism in Sports Nutrition." Driskell, J. & Wolnsky, I. Eds. CRC Press. Boca Raton, FL. (2000).

[7] S.J. Nechuta, B.J. Caan, W.Y. Chen, W.Y. Lu, Z. Chen. "Soy Food Intake After Diagnosis of Breast Cancer and Survival: An In-Depth Analysis of

Combined Evidence From Cohort Studies of U.S. and Chinese Women." *The American Journal of Clinical Nutrition.* 96(1) (2012): 123-132.

[8] B.J. Caan, L. Natarajan, B. Parker, et. al. "Soy Food Consumption and Breast Cancer Prognosis." *Cancer Epidemiology Biomarkers and Prevention.* 20(5) (2011): 854-858.

[9] M.L. Garg, L.G. Wood, H. Singh, & P.J. Moughan. "Means of Delivering Recommended Levels of Long Chain n-3 Polyunsaturated Fatty Acids in Human Diets." *Journal of Food Science.* 71(5) (2006): R66-R71.

[10] L.K. Stamp, et. al. "Diet and Rheumatoid Arthritis: A Review of the Literature." *Seminars in Arthritis.* 35 (2005): 77-94.

[11] J.K. Chan, B.E. McDonald, J.M. Gerrard, V.M. Bruce, B.J. Weaver, & B.J. Holub. "Effect of Dietary Alpha-Linoleic Acid and its Ratio to Linoleic Acid on Platelet and Plasma Fatty Acids and Thermogenesis." *Lipids.* 28(9) (1993): 811-817.

[12] F.B. Hu, J.E. Manson, & W.C. Willett. "Types of Dietary Fat and Risk of Coronary Heart Disease: A Critical Review." *Journal of the American College of Nutrition.* 20(1) (2001): 5-19.

[13] Y. Mineharu, A. Kiozumi, Y. Wada, H. Iso, Y. Watanabe, et. al. "Coffee, Green Tea, Black Tea, and Oolong Tea Consumption and Risk of Mortality from Cardiovascular Disease in Japanese Men and Women." *Journal of Epidemiology and Community Health.* 65 (2011): 230-240.

[14] D. Conen, S.E. Chiuve, B.M. Everett, S.M. Zhang, J.E. Buring, & C.M. Albert. "Caffeine Consumption and Incident Atrial Fibrillation in Women." The *American Journal of Clinical Nutrition.* 92(3) (2010): 509-514.

[15] A.E. Mesas, L.M. Leon-Muñoz, F. Rodriquez-Artalejo, & E. Lopez-Garcia. "The Effect of Coffee on Blood Pressure and Cardiovascular Disease in Hypertensive Individuals: A Systematic Review and Meta-Analysis." *The American Journal of Clinical Nutrition.* 94(4) (2011): 1113-1126.

[16] M.G. Silletta, R. Marfisi, G. Levantesi, A. Boccanelli, C. Chieffo, et. al. "Coffee Consumption and Risk of Cardiovascular Events after Acute Myocardial Infarction." *Circulation.* 116 (2007): 2944-2951.

[17] W. Zhang, E. Lopez-Garcia, T.Y. Li, F.B. Hu, & R.M. Van Dam. "Coffee Consumption and Risk of Cardiovascular Diseases and All-Cause Mortality Among Men with Type 2 Diabetes." *Diabetes Care.* 32(6) (2009): 1043-1045.

[18] E. Lopez-Garcia, R.M. Van Dam, W.C. Willett, E.B. Rimm, J.E. Manson, et. al. "Coffee Consumption and Coronary Heart Disease in Men and Women." *Circulation.* 113 (2006): 2045-2053.

[19] D.E. Grobbee, E.B. Rimm, E. Giovannucci, G. Colditz, M. Stampfer, et. al. "Coffee, Caffeine, and Cardiovascular Disease in Men." *New England Journal of Medicine.* 323 (1990): 1026-1032.

[20] D.C. Frankenfield, E.R. Muth, W.A. Rowe. "The Harris-Benedict Studies of Human Basal Metabolism: History and Limitations." *Journal of the American Dietetic Association.* 98 (1998): 439-445.

[21] D.R. Taaffe, J. Thompson, G. Butterfield, R. Marcus. "Accuracy of Equations to Predict Basal Metabolic Rate in Older Women." *Journal of the American Dietetic Association.* 95 (1995):1387-1392.

[22] F.F. Samaha, N. Iqbal, P. Seshadri, K.L., Chicano, D. Daily, J. McGrory, et. al. "A Low-Carbohydrate as Compared with a Low-Fat Diet in Severe Obesity." *New England Journal of Medicine.* 348 (2003): 2074-2081.

[23] D.M. Bravata, L. Sanders, J. Huang, H.M. Krumholz, I. Olkin, C.D. Gardner, et. al."Efficacy and Safety of Low-Carbohydrate Diets." *Journal of the American Medical Association.* 289(14) (2003): 1837-1850.

[24] A.B. Natow, & J. Heslin. *The Most Complete Food Counter.* New York: Pocket Books, 1999.

[25] D.K. Layman, J.E. Erickson, H. Shiue, C.T. Sather, & J. Baumt. "Increased Dietary Protein Modifies Glucose and Insulin Homeostasis in Adult

Women During Weight Loss." *The Journal of Nutrition*. 133 (2003): 405-410.

[26] N.R. Rodriguez, & P.C. Gaine. "Get the Essentials: Protein in the Diets of Healthy, Physically Active Men and Women." *ACSM's Health and Fitness Journal*. 11(2) (2007): 13-17.

[27] M.L. Butryn, S. Phelan, J.O. Hill, & R.R. Wing. "Consistent Self-Monitoring of Weight: A Key Component of Successful Weight Loss Maintenance." *Obesity*. 15 (2007): 3091-3096.

Chapter 14

[1] A.M. Miniño, S.L. Murphy, J. Xu, & K.D. Kochanek. "Deaths: Final data for 2008 [PDF-2.9M]. *National Vital Statistics Reports*; vol. 59 no 10." Hyattsville, MD: National Center for Health Statistics. (2011).

[2] J.S. Schiller, et. al.

[3] American Heart Association. "Two Steps to Staying Alive with Hands-Only™ CPR." 2012.< http://www.heart.org/HEARTORG/CPRAndECC/HandsOnlyCPR/Hands-Only-CPR_UCM_440559_SubHomePage.jsp > (16 September 2012).

[4] B.J. Bobrow, D.W. Spaite, R.A. Berg, U. Stolz, A.B. Sanders, et. al. "Chest Compression-Only CPR by Lay Rescuers and Survival from Out-of-Hospital Cardiac Arrest." *Journal of the American Medical Association*. 304(13) (2010): 1447-1454.

Appendix 1

Mike's Story

Mike was 44 years old when he suffered his heart attack in March 2007. He had a 100% blockage of his left anterior descending artery, which caused symptoms while vacationing in Puerto Rico. This resulted in an angioplasty with two stents. Here is his story:

The Young Buck

How I Spent My 2007 Spring Vacation

Friday was the big day when Julie, Jose, and I were headed for the rainforest in Puerto Rico, followed by Vieques Island – the most spectacular luminescent bays in the world. Julie and Jose are two of my dear friends who had persuasively talked me into vacationing with them and wouldn't take no for an answer. I guess this was their effort to cheer me up after losing my long-term love three weeks prior. It was a difficult breakup which felt more like a divorce. Our plan on this particular Friday was to hike in the rainforest, hitch a plane ride over to the island, take out the kayaks, and then go swimming. That was the idea.

We arrived at the rainforest at about one o'clock. Julie stayed in the car because of sore feet. Jose and I started walking the rainforest, admiring this lush green, with parrots and banana and palm trees surrounding us. I immediately began taking photographs of the trees and roots that caught my eye. It was truly magnificent!

As we started walking up a cobblestone path, I started to notice an uncomfortable feeling in my windpipe as I took each breath. I had remarked to Jose that something didn't feel right. Knowing my history of anxiety, he asked, "How long has it been since you had a panic attack?"

"It's been many, many years," I replied. "That's not what this is. This is definitely something, but I don't know what. I'm thinking it might be my stomach."

We continued walking a little further, as I began feeling more and more uneasy, with an ache and pressure in my chest. "I think I better go back down," I said. When we finally arrived to our car, I told him, "If I were back in the States, I'd be on my way to the hospital."

He took that statement quite seriously and quickly started looking for help. While driving on the highway toward the city, I begged him to stop at a roadside souvenir shop to pick up one more rainforest mug and see if they carried any aspirin. By now, I felt sick to my stomach.

I was in no luck with the aspirin, so just ended up taking some Alka Seltzer and a Klonopin˙ tablet to calm my nerves, as we continued on our journey. A couple of miles further down the highway, I insisted Jose pull over to the side where I immediately threw up. Further on, we saw a cop car with flashing lights by the side of the road. Jose stopped and explained what was going on to the officer, who directed us to a small hospital in Fajardo, the eastern region of Puerto Rico which borders the Atlantic Ocean.

The hospital was a rather small, non-descript building. Once inside, the receptionist took quite a bit of time to get me in. She was well aware of my chest pains, but kept saying, "Somebody's coming." It was just like there was no urgency about it ... until reading my EKG. Although it seemed like forever, it was probably only 20 minutes.

"Michael," the doctor said, "you may be in the middle of a serious coronary incident." His appearance was striking, with silvery gray hair and beard, speaking with a thick Hispanic accent. "You are not going anywhere," he added. I requested my cousin Richard be called. Afterwards, they could do whatever they had to with me. Jose did the honors of calling Richard, saying I had experienced a severe heart attack and that he'd call back when he had more information.

The next several hours were a blur. They put me on a gurney, wheeled me into a trauma room, and rather forcefully inserted a urinary catheter – the worst part of the whole experience. I wasn't thinking clearly after this point. I don't know what state of consciousness I had shifted into, but my frame of mind was awfully foggy. The morphine they shot me full of may have had something to do with that.

It still never occurred to me that something untoward was about to happen. I figured, people have heart attacks; go to the hospital; clot-busting drugs are given to open the blockages and the issue is resolved. The problem was they couldn't open up the clot. They really thinned my blood down to the point where taking blood out of my arm from a little pin prick resulted in continuous bleeding for about an hour! I had no clotting at all. They just thinned my blood down to nothing. "You know there's a danger of bleeding in your brain," the doctor said. I replied, "Whatever ... whatever."

"We're going to stabilize you before sending you to a hospital with cardiac capabilities," they said. "We'll helicopter you to the hospital in San Pablo where a surgical team will be waiting for you." They wanted to take me in the helicopter because of time and distance. Too much time had already passed.

The helicopter was in the hospital parking lot with the paramedics waiting for an ambulance to bring me over. The distance from the ambulance to chopper was only a few hundred feet. Julie remarked that they could have easily wheeled me out, but it's protocol that you be taken by ambulance. So when the ambulance arrived, I was wheeled backwards down these hallways with my head in the direction we were moving. I felt as if I was being abducted by a UFO due to the lights I kept seeing passing over me. It all seemed so unreal.

When I finally arrived at the Hospital Hima San Pablo-Bayamon, the medical team was getting prepped in the catheterization lab, and anxiously had me sign a whole bunch of waivers about the risk of puncturing an artery and death. Once the papers were signed, it wasn't long before the cardiologist started the catheterization. At one point, he said, "This is very bad. The artery is significantly clogged and full of plaque. This is going to be very difficult, but we have some options." He never said what they were, but I quickly replied, "Just go for it."

They told me I could die, among other potential effects. All along it didn't feel that serious to me. You can be really sick with something and feel like you're going to die. I didn't really feel this overwhelming sickness.

The procedures performed were a left heart catheterization, a left ventriculogram, and a percutaneous transluminal coronary angioplasty (PTCA) with stents. Apparently it took a lot longer than the cardiologist had anticipated. After the procedures, he asked if the pain was gone.

"Yes," I said.

"Okay, we're all set. We can go."

I was kind of joking with him and started getting off the gurney.

"No, no! Not you! Everybody else can go."

It was an immediate response on my part, and I guess I was kind of joking around too. I think I was just in shock.

At the time, I was completely unaware of just how fragile my condition really was. What the cardiologist told Jose was that I could die at any time. Jose passed this information back to my family in the States as sensitively as he could. "So he's out of surgery and he's all right?" my cousin asked. "No, that's not what I'm trying to tell you! Things are not going as well as could be," Jose replied. Later, I understood the tremendous relief in my cousin Richard's voice when I finally spoke with him the following day.

Another doctor came to my room the next morning and said, "I expected you to be in heart failure this morning." "Was there heart damage?" I asked. "Extensive," was his reply. "Will I be able to ride my bicycle?" I asked. "In the future," he answered. At this point, I'm thinking, "Do you have any good news?" "I want you to rest today," he said. "I don't want you moving around much. We need to get you stabilized. You had what we call a 'widow-maker.'" I later learned that this is a specific kind of heart attack in which the left anterior descending artery gets blocked, shutting off blood flow to the left side of your heart, which is where the largest volume of blood is pumped throughout the body. Apparently, the first 24 hours are the most critical.

My four years of high school Spanish would allow me to ask where the bathroom, school, library and house are, but that's about it. I remember during my first morning in the ICU, my nurse, Maria, brought me a frothy milk substance with a glass of water. She was warm and friendly, with a mischievous gleam in her eyes. I think she said "medicina" or something, and I thought I was supposed to drink it. Like a good patient, I picked up the plastic cup and drank what turned out to be mouthwash. When she returned and realized what I had done, we both had a good laugh about it. That was just the beginning of communication difficulties which weren't all as comical.

When the doctor arrived the next morning, which was Sunday, he said he wanted me out of bed and to start becoming more active. I kept thinking my heart was going to stop beating and made him fully aware of these concerns. He assured me it wasn't going to happen. "We're not seeing the complications I expected, so I want you to get out of bed today and sit in a chair," he said.

Later that night, the same doctor came to my room and asked, "So did you get out of bed?" "I couldn't get out of bed. They would have to unhook me from all of these wires," I answered. "You had a heart attack; not a stroke. I want you up and moving around again," he ordered. "Depending on how you're doing, we'll discharge you either Tuesday or Wednesday," he added. This doctor was one of the few who spoke English, and was really reassuring.

Before I knew it, Tuesday had arrived. Apparently, a cardiologist was in to see me while I was asleep, and mentioned I could go home today. I had it set in my mind that there was no way I was being discharged until at least Wednesday. My flight home wasn't scheduled until later in the day on Wednesday, and there was no way I was leaving this hospital any sooner, where I wouldn't be monitored. "Get somebody in here who speaks English!" I demanded. "Jose, tell these people I'm not leaving. They can call security and drag me out of here but I'm not leaving! It's scary enough as it is. I'm staying one more day!" Luckily, an internist was there who granted me the additional day. After receiving this confirmation, I could mentally prepare for my flight home.

When I finally arrived home, Richard and my lovely cat, Skee, gave me a wonderful greeting. The phone calls started trickling in. I could now begin the mending process. I could see that it would be a long road to physical, emotional and spiritual recovery.

At first, I didn't know what I could, couldn't and shouldn't do. I was afraid to drag my garbage can to the curb or walk up my basement stairs. How would I do laundry or clean Skee's litter box? This was tough to deal with, especially since I made a habit of compulsively exercising, no matter how I felt. The times I came home exhausted from work on the hottest days of the year, I would still force myself to go out for a grueling bike ride. On the other hand, if it was a cold winter's night when arriving home, I might opt to do a fast-paced yoga workout. The point is I was always highly active.

My experience with exercise began in my early 20s, when I ate junk food and smoked a pack of cigarettes a day. A buddy sold me a bicycle for $5, which I decided to ride to work one day. I arrived at work shaking and nauseous, despite the fact that the ride was only a flat couple of miles. Seeing how out-of-shape I was, a few friends convinced me to join a local health spa. Even though I continued to smoke, I was amazed to see how rapidly my endurance improved. At 5'7, 148 lbs, and not much body fat to brag about, I had always been a skinny weakling. But since I started exercising at the spa, I started seeing increases in muscular size, strength and definition. Upon seeing an old high school acquaintance who picked on me back then, I became hooked on exercise after he remarked, "Wow, you really filled out!"

After a couple of years of being nagged by friends and co-workers, I finally threw away the pack of cigarettes and never looked back. I had experienced yet another triumph! It was elating, seeing what exercise could do for me and how good it felt; both physically and emotionally.

Shortly after this event, I was so afraid I would do something to hurt my heart again. I felt no amount of reassurance would quell that fear. Should I simply accept the notion that the physically fit and confident person I had become died in Puerto Rico?

Nutrition was another big concern for me. Prior to my heart attack, I was aware that my cholesterol was high, despite eating a relatively low fat diet. I would look at labels and try to pick foods lower in saturated fat, in particular. Looking back, I realize I ate a lot of frozen dinners and snacked on a lot of chips. Despite coming from the health food section of the stores, they came with a lot of fat and preservatives. I also had the habit of "letting myself go" several times a week where I would eat anything – ice cream, fried eggs, etc. Now that I'm back home, how do I eat to prevent another attack?

After a few weeks of my living in fear at home, my cardiologist referred me to a cardiac rehab program at my local hospital. With exercise being an important part of my life for so long, I was eager to get back, yet scared to death! I definitely had some mixed emotions bottled up inside. Nevertheless, I followed doctor's orders and joined the program.

My first appointment with the rehab staff was simply to meet them and tour the impressive facility. They had a wide variety of aerobic equipment, including bikes, treadmills, rowing machines and elliptical walkers. The resistance training equipment was not too shabby either. It was made up of dumbbells ranging from a single pound to 60 pounds! A colorful array of resistance bands were also hanging around, in addition to stability balls and exercise mats. I was like a kid in a candy store.

My next visit was the real deal. After an informative lecture on matters of the heart, I pasted EKG electrodes on my chest, strapped on my heart monitor and went to work in the exercise room. The nurse and exercise physiologist guided me on the proper use of the machine of my choice and explained how intense the exercise should be. After 45 minutes of aerobic exercise, we moved to the weight room for strength training. Although I was still cautious, it was great to finally be exercising again. Having competent medical professionals by my side made all the difference.

I was very consistent with my attendance in cardiac rehab. It was no time before I began pushing myself harder with aerobics and using heavier dumbbells for weight training. In fact, the nurse in charge wanted me to slow down! I obeyed … but just a little. Although I started riding my bike again, I always monitored my heart rate and kept it in the range prescribed by my cardiologist. I did no riding in the deep woods and always carried a cell phone. I remained cautious.

Now at the three-year mark, I am working out harder than I thought I would ever be able to. A stress test in September 2007 showed I was able to exercise to a level of 14.5 METs. I learned from the rehab staff that METs stands for "metabolic equivalents," and tells how much of the oxygen I breathe in my body is utilizing. Apparently 14.5 METs represents my maximum. For general aerobic exercise, I've built myself up to maintain 9 METs for 30 to 60 minutes. This would be equivalent to performing heavy snow-shoveling or fast stair-climbing. My heart rate and blood pressures have tolerated this extremely well.

Regarding nutrition, cardiac rehab has educated me on how to structure my diet for both heart health and exercise performance. I've increased my consumption of fruits, vegetables and whole grains, while cutting out excess simple sugars, fried food and red meat. I've learned healthy alternatives to the unhealthy snacks I'd binged on for so many years. I now have structure in my diet, which has given me more structure in my life in general.

The hardest part about having sustained heart damage in an otherwise athletic body has been the fear that I would be unable to sustain the vigorous exercise routines I've engaged in prior to the attack. I admit to pushing myself in unhealthy ways and ignoring the overwhelming amount of stress I was under. Through my involvement in the cardiac rehab program, I have learned that both mind and body must be cared for in an ongoing manner. Furthermore, I've learned how to eat and exercise in a fashion tailored to my personal goals. I wholeheartedly believe I've achieved a level of overall health that actually surpasses my former self.

Appendix 2

Sample Exercise Log

Date: Mon, 7/2/12 **Time:** 2pm **Workout:** Chest & Back **Bodyweight:** 200lbs

Cardio: Treadmill, 45min @ 6am, Speed: 3.7mph Incline: 10%,

Heart Rate Range: 130-140bpm

EXERCISE	SET #1 WEIGHT LIFTED/# OF REPETITIONS	SET#2	SET#3	SET#4
Dumbbell chest press on Swiss ball	40lbs/15x	65lbs/15x	90lbs/12x	100lbs/10x
Reverse-grip cable pulldown (blue theraband tubing)	15x	15x	15x	15x
Dumbbell fly on Swiss ball	25lbs/15x	35lbs/15x	45lbs/12x	50lbs/11x
Bent over dumbbell row	40lbs/15x	60lbs/13x	80lbs/10z	80lbs/10x
Kneeling cable pullover (green theraband tubing)	15x	15x	15x	15x
Dumbbell upright row	20lbs/15x	30lbs/15x	40lbs/13x	50lbs/10x
Swiss ball back extension	15x	15x	15x	15x

Appendix 3

Sample Exercise Log (Blank)

Date: ___ Time: ____ Workout: ___ Bodyweight: _____

Cardio: _____

Heart Rate Range: _____

EXERCISE	SET #1 WEIGHT LIFTED/# OF REPETITIONS	SET#2	SET#3	SET#4

Appendix 4

Sample Weight Loss Diet (140 pound female)

MEAL NO.1	**CAL**	**FAT**	**CARBS**	**PROTEIN**
4 egg whites	68	0	0	16
½ cup oatmeal	150	3	27	5
1 apple w/ cinnamon	80	1	18	0
Total:	*298*	*4*	*45*	*21*

MEAL NO.2	**CAL**	**FAT**	**CARBS**	**PROTEIN**
1 scoop whey isolate	100	0	0	25
1 cup almond milk	60	2.5	8	1
1 cup strawberries	52	0	14	1
1.5 cups ↑fiber cereal	220	3	46	4
Total:	*432*	*5.5*	*68*	*31*

MEAL NO.3	**CAL**	**FAT**	**CARBS**	**PROTEIN**
3oz. boneless skinless chicken breast	130	2	0	27
6oz. sweet potato	200	1	48	1
1 cup broccoli	30	0	4	1
Total:	*360*	*3*	*52*	*29*

MEAL NO.4	CAL	FAT	CARBS	PROTEIN
2 slices Ezekiel bread	160	1	30	8
2 Tbsp. all-natural peanut butter	180	15	6	8
Total:	**340**	**16**	**36**	**16**

MEAL NO.5	CAL	FAT	CARBS	PROTEIN
3oz. salmon	183	9	0	23
¾ cup brown rice	150	0	35	3
2 cups green salad with 1 Tbsp. olive oil and balsamic vinegar	140	14	3	1
Total	*473*	*23*	*38*	*27*

Daily Total Calories = 1903

Daily Total Grams of Fat = 52

Daily Total grams of Carbohydrates = 239

Daily Total Grams of Protein = 124

52 grams of fat * 9 calories = 468 calories from fat
468 calories from fat / 1903 total calories = 0.246 or **25% calories from fat**
239 grams of carbs * 4 calories = 956 calories from carbs
956 calories from carbs / 1903 total calories = 0.502 or **50% calories from carbs**
124 grams of protein * 4 calories = 496 calories from protein
496 calories from protein / 1903 total calories = 0.261 or **25% calories from protein**

Appendix 5

Sample Weight Maintenance Diet (185 pound male)

MEAL No.1	CAL	FAT	CARBS	PROTEIN
1 scoop whey protein isolate(in water)	100	0	0	25
1 cup oatmeal (not instant)	300	6	54	10
1 sliced apple with cinnamon	80	1	18	0
¼ cup walnuts	200	20	4	3
Total:	**680**	**27**	**76**	**38**

MEAL No.2	CAL	FAT	CARBS	PROTEIN
4oz. can of tuna (in water)with 2 Tbsp. salsa	130	2	2	26
¾ cup brown rice	150	0	35	3
2/3 cup corn (fresh or frozen)	100	1	20	3
Total:	**380**	**3**	**57**	**32**

MEAL No.3	CAL	FAT	CARBS	PROTEIN
1 pear	100	1	25	1
2 slices Ezekiel bread	160	1	30	8
3oz. ground turkey	100	3	0	19
4oz. 2% low-fat cottage cheese	101	2	4	16
Total:	**461**	**7**	**59**	**44**

MEAL NO.4	CAL	FAT	CARBS	PROTEIN
1.5 cups brown rice	300	0	70	6
1 cup cooked lima beans	188	0	36	12
4.5oz. asparagus	20	0	0	2
Total:	**508**	**0**	*106*	**20**

MEAL NO.5	CAL	FAT	CARBS	PROTEIN
2 scoops whey protein isolate (in water)	200	0	0	50
2 Tbsp. flax seed oil	240	28	0	0
1 Tbsp. all-natural peanut butter	90	7	3	4
Total:	*530*	*35*	*3*	*54*

Daily Total Calories = 2559

Daily Total Grams of Fat = 72

Daily Total grams of Carbohydrates = 301

Daily Total Grams of Protein = 188

72 grams of fat * 9 calories = 648 calories from fat
648 calories from fat / 2559 total calories = 0.253 or **25% calories from fat**
301 grams of carbs * 4 calories = 1204 calories from carbs
1204 calories from carbs / 2559 total calories = 0.47 or **47% calories from carbs**
188 grams of protein * 4 calories = 752 calories from protein
752 calories from protein / 2559 total calories = 0.294 or **29% calories from protein**

Appendix 6

Medication List

Name:_____ Date of Birth:_____

Address:_____ Phone #:_____

City:_____ State:_____ Zip:_____

Immunization Record (Record the date and year of last dose taken):

Tetanus:_____ Hepatitis Vaccine:_____

Flu Vaccine:_____ Pneumonia Vaccine:_____

Other:_____

Allergies (Name your allergies and describe your reaction):

List all medications you are currently taking. Include prescription and over-the-counter medications, dietary supplements and medications taken "as needed" (such as nitroglycerin).

DATE STARTED	NAME OF MED	DOSE/DIRECTIONS	DATE STOPPED	NOTES: REASON FOR TAKING; NAME OF DOCTOR

DATE STARTED	NAME OF MED	DOSE/DIRECTIONS	DATE STOPPED	NOTES: REASON FOR TAKING; NAME OF DOCTOR

Resources *

Academy of Nutrition and Dietetics
120 South Riverside Plaza, Suite 2000
Chicago, IL 60606
www.eatright.org
The best source for accurate, credible and timely food and nutrition information. It is committed to improving the nation's health and advancing the profession of dietetics through research, education and advocacy.

American Association of Cardiovascular and Pulmonary Rehabilitation
330 N. Wabash Avenue, Suite 2000
Chicago, IL 60611
www.aacvpr.org
National Association whose mission is to reduce morbidity, mortality and disability from cardiovascular and pulmonary disease through education, prevention, rehabilitation research and disease management.

American College of Sports Medicine
401 West Michigan Street
Indianapolis, IN 46202
www.acsm.org
The largest sports medicine and exercise science organization in the world, with over 45,000 members and certified professionals worldwide. It is dedicated to advancing and integrating scientific research to provide education and practical applications of exercise science and sports medicine.

American Heart Association
7272 Greenville Avenue
Dallas, TX 75231
www.heart.org
The leading organization to promote funding for research and education with the goal of building healthier lives, free of cardiovascular disease and stroke.

Centers for Disease Control and Prevention

---

* Please note: The accuracy of the listings above cannot be guaranteed as websites, agencies, and associations may change or cease operation. Furthermore, the above listing does not imply endorsements of any kind.

1600 Clifton Road
Atlanta, GA 30333
www.cdc.gov
The CDC's mission is to promote health and quality of life by preventing and controlling disease, injury and disability.

Exercise is Medicine
401 West Michigan Street
Indianapolis, IN 46202
www.exerciseismedicine.org
A branch of the American College of Sports Medicine with the goal to improve public health and reduce health care costs by making physical activity and exercise a standard part of global disease prevention and treatment medical paradigm.

Gatorade Sports Science Institute
617 West Main Street
Barrington, IL 60010
www.gssiweb.com
A leading organization which provides up-to-date research and education in hydration and nutrition science.

Health Journeys
891 Moe Drive, Suite C
Akron, OH 44310-2538
Resources for mind, body and spirit.
www.healthjourneys.com

European Heart Network
Rue Montoyer 31
1000 Brussels
Belgium
www.ehnheart.org
A leading organization with 33 members in 26 European countries. Members are national heart foundations and other non-governmental heart-health organizations committed to prevention of cardiovascular disease in Europe.

Heart and Stroke Foundation of Canada
222 Queen Street, Suite 1402

Ottawa, ON K1P 5V9

www.heartandstroke.com

A volunteer-based health charity which leads in eliminating heart disease and stroke and reducing their impact through advocacy, the advancement of research and its application, and the promotion of healthy living.

British Heart Foundation
Greater London House
180 Hampstead Road
London
NW1 7AW

www.bhf.org.uk

A charity-based organization aimed to help fund research and education to support those living with heart disease, ensure quality of care, and reduce morbidity and mortality associated with cardiovascular disease.

To provide you with the most up-to-date information within the fields of exercise science and medicine, here are some valuable and credible resources:

MedlinePlus – A service of the U.S. National Library of Medicine and National Institutes of Health. The Drugs and Supplements tab will enable you to access information on a comprehensive listing of medications and supplements as well as their actions, potential side effects, and interactions. It is a trusted source of health information and can be accessed at: http://www.nlm.nih.gov/medlineplus/druginformation.html.

Lab Tests Online – A peer-reviewed, non-commercial, and patient-centered public resource on clinical laboratory testing from the professionals who actually do the testing. It can be accessed at: http://labtestsonline.org.

Exercise Prescription on the Internet – A free resource for the exercise professional, coach, or fitness enthusiast featuring comprehensive exercise libraries, fitness assessment calculators, and reference articles. The content of this website is also available on CD-ROM. It can be accessed at: http://exrx.net.

Bibliography

American College of Sports Medicine. *ACSM's Exercise Management for Persons with Chronic Diseases and Disabilities.* Champaign, IL: Human Kinetics, 1997.

American Heart Association. "Doctors Should Encourage Cardiac Rehab Programs." 2005. < http://newsroom.heart.org/news/doctors-should-encourage-cardiac-223005 > Accessed March 6, 2006.

American Heart Association. "Two Steps to Staying Alive with Hands-Only™ CPR." 2012.< http://www.heart.org/HEARTORG/CPRAndECC/HandsOnlyCPR/Hands-Only-CPR_UCM_440559_SubHomePage.jsp > (16 September 2012)

Baechle, T.R. & Earle, R. (Eds.). *Essentials of Strength Training and Conditioning* (2nd ed.). Champaign, IL: Human Kinetics, 2000.

Bravata, D.M., Sanders, L., Huang, J., Krumholz, H.M., Olkin, I., Gardner, C.D., et al. "Efficacy and Safety of Low-Carbohydrate Diets." *Journal of the American Medical Association.* 289(14) (2003): 1837-1850.

Bobrow, B.J., Spaite, D.W., Berg, R.A., Stolz, U., Sanders, A.B., et al. "Chest Compression-Only CPR by Lay Rescuers and Survival from Out-of-Hospital Cardiac Arrest." *Journal of the American Medical Association.* 304(13) (2010): 1447-1454.

Butryn, M.L., Phelan, S., Hill, J.O., & Wing, R.R. "Consistent Self-Monitoring of Weight: A Key Component of Successful Weight Loss Maintenance." *Obesity.* 15 (2007): 3091-3096.

Bucci, L.R., & Unlu, L. "Protein and Amino Acids in Exercise and Sport." In: "Energy-Yielding Macronutrients and Energy Metabolism in Sports Nutrition." Driskell, J. & Wolnsky, I. Eds. CRC Press. Boca Raton, FL. (2000).

Centers for Disease Control and Prevention (CDC). "Prevalence and Most Common Causes of Disability among Adults – United States, 2005." *Morbidity and Mortality Weekly Report.* 58 (2009): 421-426.

Chan, J.K., McDonald, B.E., Gerrard, J.M., Bruce, V.M., Weaver, B.J., & Holub, B. J. "Effect of Dietary Alpha-Linoleic Acid and its Ratio to Linoleic Acid on Platelet and Plasma Fatty Acids and Thermogenesis." *Lipids.* 28(9) (1993): 811-817.

Caan, B.J., Natarajan, L., Parker, B., et. al. "Soy Food Consumption and Breast Cancer Prognosis." *Cancer Epidemiology Biomarkers and Prevention.* 20 (5) (2011): 854-858.

Conen, D., Chiuve, S.E., Everett, B.M., Zhang, S.M., Buring, J.E., & Albert, C.M. "Caffeine Consumption and Incident Atrial Fibrillation in Women." *The American Journal of Clinical Nutrition.* 92(3) (2010): 509-514.

Cox, J.L., Ad, N., Palazzo, T., Fitzpatrick, S., Suyderhoud, J.P., DeGroot, K.W., et al. "Current Status of the Maze Procedure for the Treatment of Atrial Fibrillation." *Seminars of Thoracic and Cardiovascular Surgery.* 12(1) (2000): 15-19.

Cummins, R.O. (Ed.). *ACLS Provider Manual.* Dallas, TX: American Heart Association. (2001).

Daubenmier, J.J., Weidner, G., Sumner, M., Mendell, N., Merritt-Worden, T., Studley, J., et al. "The Contribution of Changes in Diet, Exercise, and Stress Management to Changes in Coronary Risk in Women and Men in the Multisite Cardiac Lifestyle Intervention Program." *Annals of Behavioral Medicine.* 33(1) (2007): 57-68.

Davidson, K.W., et al. "Assessment and Treatment of Depression in Patients with Cardiovascular Disease: National Heart, Lung, and Blood Institute Working Group Report." *Psychosomatic Medicine.* 68(5) (2006): 645-650.

"Financial Preparedness Critical to Heart Disease Sufferers." Council For Disability Awareness. June, 2008. <

http://www.disabilitycanhappen.org/chances_disability/causes.asp > (12 August 2012).

Frankenfield, D.C., Muth, E.R., Rowe, W.A. "The Harris-Benedict Studies of Human Basal Metabolism: History and Limitations." *Journal of the American Dietetic Association.* 98 (1998): 439-445.

Gabriel, R., Alonso, M., Reviriego, B., Muñiz, J., Vega, S., et.al. "Ten-Year Fatal and Non-Fatal Myocardial Infarction Incidence in Elderly Populations in Spain: The Epicardian Cohort Study." *Biomed Central Public Health.* 9 (2009): 360.

Garg, M.L., Wood, L.G., Singh, H., & Moughan, P.J. "Means of Delivering Recommended Levels of Long Chain n-3 Polyunsaturated Fatty Acids in Human Diets." *Journal of Food Science.* 71(5) (2006): R66-R71.

Gellish, R.L., Goslin, B.R., Olson, R.E., McDonald, A., Russi, G.D., & Moudgil, V.K. "Longitudinal Modeling of the Relationship Between Age and Maximal HeartRate." Medicine and Science in Sports and Exercise. 39(5) (2007): 822-829.

Girlanda, P., Dattola, R., Venuto, C., Mangiapane, R., Nicolosi, C., & Messina, C. "Local Steroid Treatment in Idiopathic Carpal Tunnel Syndrome: Short-and Long-Term Efficacy." *Journal of Neurology.* 240(3) (1993): 187-190.

Go, A.S., Mozaffarian, D., Roger, V.L., Benjamin, E.J., Berry, J.D., et. al. AHA Statistical Update. "Heart Disease and Stroke Statistics – 2013 Update." Circulation. 2013. < http://circ.ahajournals.org/content/127/1/e6.full> Accessed January 7, 2013. doi: 10.1161/CIR.obo13e31828124ad.

Grobbee, D.E., Rimm, E.B., Giovannucci, E., Colditz, G., Stampfer, et al. "Coffee, Caffeine, and Cardiovascular Disease in Men." *New England Journal of Medicine.* 323 (1990): 1026-1032.

Haskell, W.L., Lee, I., Pate, R.R., Powell, K.E., Blair, S.N., Franklin, B.A., et al. "Physical Activity and Public Health: Updated Recommendation for Adults from The American College of Sports Medicine and the American

Heart Association." *Medicine and Science in Sports and Exercise.* 39(8) (2007): 1423-1434.

Hauser, A. "30 Minutes of Exercise Does the Trick, Study Says." *Everyday Health.* 2012. <http://www.everydayhealth.com/fitness/0824/30-minutes-of-exercise-does-the-trick-study-says.aspx?xid=aol_eh-genvid_5_20120827_&aolcat=HLT&icid=maing-grid10%7Chtmlws-main-bb%7Cdl36%7Csec1_lnk3%26pLid%3D197614> (28 August 2012).

Heaney, R.P. "Protein and Calcium: Antagonists or Synergists?" *The American Journal of Clinical Nutrition.* 75(4) (2002): 609-610.

Hew, T.D., Chorley, J.N., Cianca, J.C., & Divine, J.G. "The Incidence, Risk Factors, and Clinical Manifestations of Hyponatremia in Marathon Runners." *Clinical Journal of Sports Medicine.* 13 (2003): 41-47.

Hu, F.B., Manson, J.E., & Willett, W.C. "Types of Dietary Fat and Risk of Coronary Heart Disease: A Critical Review." *Journal of the American College of Nutrition.* 20(1) (2001): 5-19.

Hurst, W. *The Heart, Arteries, and Veins* (10th ed.). New York, NY: McGraw-Hill, 2002.

Juurlink, D.N., Tu, J.V., & Mamdani, M.M. "Interactions Between Clopidogrel and Proton Pump Inhibitors." *Canadian Medical Association Journal.* 180(12) (2009): 1229.

Kaminsky, L.A., Bonzheim, K.A., Garber, C.E., Glass, S.C., Hamm, L.F., Kohl III, H.W., & Mikesky, A. (Eds.). *ACSM's Resource Manual for Guidelines for Exercise Testing and Prescription* (4th Ed.). Baltimore: Lippincott Williams &Wilkins, 2006.

Kripalani, L.S., Roumie, L.C., Dalal, K.A., Cawthon, C., Businger, A., et al. "Effect of a Pharmacist Intervention on Clinically Important Medication Errors After Hospital Discharge: A Randomized Trial." *Annals of Internal Medicine.* 157(1) (2012): 1-10.

Layman, D.K., Erickson, J.E., Shiue, H., Sather, C.T., & Baumt, J. "Increased Dietary Protein Modifies Glucose and Insulin Homeostasis in Adult Women During Weight Loss." *The Journal of Nutrition*. 133 (2003): 405-410.

Lewis, S.M., Heitkemper, M.M., & Dirksen, S.R. *Medical-Surgical Nursing: Assessment and Management of Clinical Problems* (6th ed.). St. Louis, MI: Mosby, Inc., 2004.

Lopez-Garcia, E., Van Dam, R.M., Willett, W.C., Rimm, E.B., Manson, J.E., et al. "Coffee Consumption and Coronary Heart Disease in Men and Women." *Circulation*. 113 (2006): 2045-2053.

Low, P.P.L., Rutherford, K.J., Gill, H.S., & Cross, M.L. "Effects of Dietary Whey Protein Concentrate on Primary and Secondary Antibody Responses in Immunized BALB/c Mice." *International Immunopharmacology*. 3 (2003): 393-401.

Melville, N.A. "Sedentary Behavior Associated with Higher Mortality." 2011. *American College of Sports Medicine* (ACSM) 58th Annual Meeting. *Abstract 623*. Presented June 2, 2011.

Mesas, A.E., Leon-Muñoz, L.M., Rodriquez-Artalejo, F., & Lopez-Garcia, E. "The Effect of Coffee on Blood Pressure and Cardiovascular Disease in Hypertensive Individuals: A Systematic Review and Meta-Analysis." *The American Journal of Clinical Nutrition*. 94(4) (2011): 1113-1126.

Mineharu, Y., Kiozumi, A., Wada, Y., Iso, H., Watanabe, Y., et al. "Coffee, Green Tea, Black Tea, and Oolong Tea Consumption and Risk of Mortality from Cardiovascular Disease in Japanese Men and Women." *Journal of Epidemiology and Community Health*. 65 (2011): 230-240.

Miniño AM, Murphy SL, Xu J, Kochanek KD. "Deaths: Final data for 2008 [PDF-2.9M]. *National Vital Statistics Reports*; vol 59 no 10." Hyattsville, MD: National Center for Health Statistics. (2011).

Mosby's *Nursing Drug Reference*. St.Louis, MI: Mosby, Inc., 2004.

Munn, J., Herbert, R.D., & Gandevia, S.C. "Contralateral Effects of Unilateral Resistance Training: A Meta-Analysis." *Journal of Applied Physiology*. 96 (2004): 1861-1866.

Naparstek, B. *Staying Well with Guided Imagery*. New York: Warner Books, 1994.

National Institute of Mental Health. "Depression and Heart Disease, Bethesda (MD)":National Institute of Mental Health, National Institutes of Health, US Department of Health and Human Services. 2002. (NIH Publication No. 02-5004) 4 pages. <http://www.nimh.nih.gov> (2 November 2006).

Natow, A.B. & Heslin, J. *The Most Complete Food Counter*. New York: Pocket Books, 1999.

Nechuta, S.J., Caan, B.J., Chen, W.Y., Lu, W.Y., Chen, Z. "Soy Food Intake After Diagnosis of Breast Cancer and Survival: An In-Depth Analysis of Combined Evidence From Cohort Studies of U.S. and Chinese Women." *The American Journal of Clinical Nutrition*.96(1) (2012): 123-132.

Nieman, D.C. *Exercise Testing and Prescription: A Health-Related Approach* (4th ed.). Mountain View, CA: Mayfield Publishing Company, 1999.

Nissen, E.S., & Wolski, K. "Effect of Rosiglitazone on the Risk of Myocardial Infarction and Death from Cardiovascular Causes." *New England Journal of Medicine*. 356(24) (2007): 2457-2471.

Oka, R.K., King, A.C., & Young, D.R. "Sources of Social Support as Predictors of Exercise Adherence in Women and Men Ages 50 to 65 Years." *Women's Health*. 1(2) (1995): 161-175.

"A Promising Treatment for Athletes, in Blood." 2009. <http://www.nytimes.com/2009/02/17/sports/17blood.html?pagewanted=all&_r=0 > (13 July 2011).

Quinn, T.J., Klooster, J.R., & Focht, B.C. "Two Short, Daily Activity Bouts Vs. One Long Bout: Are Health and Fitness Improvements Similar Over

Twelve and Twenty-four Weeks?" *Journal of Strength and Conditioning Research.* 20(1) (2006): 130-135.

Robertson, L., A. Rogers, A. Ewing, et al. (Eds.). *American Association of Cardiovascular and Pulmonary Rehabilitation and Secondary Prevention Programs* (4th ed.). Champaign, IL: Human Kinetics, 2004.

Rodriguez, N.R., & Gaine, P.C. "Get the Essentials: Protein in the Diets of Healthy, Physically Active Men and Women." *ACSM's Health and Fitness Journal.* 11(2) (2007): 13-17.

Roger, V.L., Go, A.S., Lloyd-Jones, D.M., Adams, R.J., Berry, J.D. "Heart Disease and Stroke Statistics – 2011 Update: A Report From the American Heart Association." *Circulation.* 123 (2010): e18-e209.

Samaha, F.F., Iqbal, N., Seshadri, P., Chicano, K.L., Daily, D., McGrory, J., et al. "A Low-Carbohydrate as Compared with a Low-Fat Diet in Severe Obesity." *New England Journal of Medicine.* 348 (2003): 2074-2081.

Schiller, J.S., Lucas, J.W., Ward, B.W., Peregoy, J.A. "Summary Health Statistics for US Adults: National Health Interview Survey, 2010. National Center for Health Statistics." *Vital Health Statistics.* 10(252) (2012): 19.

Schwarzenegger, Arnold. *Encyclopedia of Modern Bodybuilding.* New York, NY: Simon & Schuster, Inc., 1985.

Silletta, M.G., Marfisi, R., Levantesi, G., Boccanelli, A., Chieffo, C., et al. "Coffee Consumption and Risk of Cardiovascular Events after Acute Myocardial Infarction." *Circulation.* 116 (2007): 2944-2951.

Smorawinski, J., Nazar, K., Kaciuba-Uscilko, H., Kaminska, E., Cybulski, G, Kodrzycka, A., et al. "Effects of 3-Day Bed Rest on Physiological Responses to Graded Exercise in Athletes and Sedentary Men." *Journal of Applied Physiology.* 91(1) (2001): 249-257.

Soni, A. "Back Problems: Use and Expenditures for the U.S. Adult Population, 2007. Statistical Brief #289." July 2010. Agency for Healthcare Research and Quality.

<http://www.meps.ahrq.gov/mepsweb/data_files/publications/st289/stat289.pdf> (15 August 2012)

Stahl, S. & Kaufman, T. "The Efficacy of an Injection of Steroids for Medial Epicondylitis: A Prospective Study of Sixty Elbows." *The Journal of Bone and Joint Surgery.* 79 (1997): 1648-1652.

Stamp, L.K., et. al. "Diet and Rheumatoid Arthritis: A Review of the Literature." *Seminars in Arthritis.* 35 (2005): 77-94.

Stone, P.H., Gratsiansky, N.A., Blokhin, A., et al. "Antianginal Efficacy of Ranolazine when Added to Maximal Therapy with Conventional Therapy: The Efficacy of Ranolazine in Chronic Angina Trial." *Circulation.* 48 (2006): 566-575.

Strauss, J. "Research Findings on Imagery & PTSD." Preliminary findings presented at the Army's 10th Annual Force Health Protection Conference. Louisville, KY, (August 2007).

"The Surgeon General's Call to Action to Prevent and Decrease Overweight and Obesity." (2007). <http://www.surgeongeneral.gov/topics/obesity/calltoaction/fact_adolescents.htm> (2 October 2008).

Taaffe, D.R., Thompson, J., Butterfield, G., Marcus, R. "Accuracy of Equations to Predict Basal Metabolic Rate in Older Women." *Journal of the American Dietetic Association.* 95 (1995):1387-1392.

Vincent, K.R., Braith, R.W., Feldman, R.A., Magyari, P.M., Cutler, R.B., Persin, S.A., et al. "Resistance Exercise and Physical Performance in Adults Aged 60 to 83." *Journal of the American Geriatrics Society.* 50(6) (2002): 1100-1107.

Wade, C. & Tavris, C. *Invitation to Psychology.* 3rd Edition. New Jersey:Pearson Prentice Hall, 2005.

Whaley, M.H., Brubaker, P.H., & Otto, R.M. (Eds.). *ACSM's Guidelines for Exercise Testing and Prescription* (7th ed.). Baltimore: Lippincott Williams & Wilkins, 2006.

Wilmore, J.H. & Costill, D.C. *Physiology of Sport and Exercise* (2nd ed.). Champaign, IL: Human Kinetics, 1999.

Wolfe, R.R. "Protein Supplements and Exercise." *American Journal of Clinical Nutrition.* 72(suppl) (2000): 551s-7s.

Wong, C.W. & Watson, D.L. "Immunomodulatory Effects of Dietary Whey Proteins in Mice." *Journal of Dairy Research.* 62 (1995): 359-368.

"You Might Have Exercise Fever, but Is It OK to Workout When Ill?" 2008. <http://www.gadsdentimes.com/article/20080131/news/801310306/1049/lifetimes.> (6 February 2008).

Zhang, W., Lopez-Garcia, E., Li, T.Y., Hu, F.B., & Van Dam, R.M. "Coffee Consumption and Risk of Cardiovascular Diseases and All-Cause Mortality Among Men with Type 2 Diabetes." *Diabetes Care.* 32(6) (2009): 1043-1045.

Acknowledgements

There are many people I have to thank for generously donating their time as well as providing their knowledge and expertise. Without their insight, this book would not have been possible. However, I am alone responsible for the contents of this book.

First and foremost, I need to thank Michael Czwilikoski for giving me the idea, confidence and inspiration to write this book.

I must thank my patients in cardiac rehab, both past and present. They shared their stories and experiences so I could relay this information to my readers. It is true that we learn through experience. It doesn't necessarily have to be our own experiences.

I also need to thank Michael Winder for walking me through the challenging steps of writing a book proposal, forming an outline, and helping with a great deal of preliminary editing. I also need to thank Laura Miller for her contribution of initial editing. I especially need to thank Dr. Jan Yager for her acting as my primary editor, as well as her tireless efforts in helping me to fulfill my potential as a writer. I need to extend that thank you to James Mapes for wisely referring me to Dr. Yager. I also thank Peggy Barber for her proofreading expertise.

I need to give a special thanks to Jillian DiViesta, RD, PA-C, and Glenn Beloso, RPh, for diligently reviewing my nutrition and medication sections.

I thank Tara Macolino for her highly-skilled artwork throughout this book. I also need to thank Todd Ganci and Julia Gerace for their professionalism and top-quality photos. I thank Gabriella Carloni for posing as the female exerciser in those photos.

Lastly, I need to thank my mother, Mary Ann Petreycik, and my fiancée, Rowena Eden, for their ongoing love and support. Rowena's creativity and computer skills proved to be an invaluable asset.

Index

About the Author

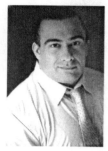

JOE PETREYCIK is a certified clinical exercise physiologist and registered nurse. He divides his time between a hospital-based cardiac rehab facility and a surgical intensive care unit in a busy inner-city hospital in southwestern Connecticut. Joe is certified as a Clinical Exercise Specialist[SM] by the American College of Sports Medicine (ACSM).

He graduated with a bachelor's degree in Exercise Science from Sacred Heart University in Fairfield, CT, where he played four years of tennis in a Division I-AA school. After working two years as an exercise physiologist, Joe continued his education at Bridgeport Hospital School of Nursing where he received his diploma in Nursing, in addition to being the sole recipient of the "Diane Avery Leadership Award and Scholarship." He immediately obtained his RN license. He has been recognized by Member of Congress Rosa L. DeLauro for his exceptional work in cardiac rehab.

Recreationally, Joe has competed at the national level as a bodybuilder in the National Physique Committee (NPC), the top amateur bodybuilding organization. He is two-time NPC Mr. CT after winning the overall title in 2008 and 2010.

Joe volunteers his time at his church as a parish nurse, where he monitors parishioners' blood pressure and addresses medically-relevant questions and concerns on a monthly basis. He also participates in the American Heart Association's Fairfield County Heart Walk, which takes place annually in southwestern Connecticut. The money raised from the event is used to fund research and educational programs for the American Heart Association.

Joe intends to utilize his education and experience as a clinical exercise physiologist, registered nurse and competitive bodybuilder who has managed to successfully lose 60 pounds, to help as many individuals as possible to reduce and eliminate as many risk factors as possible, related to our number one killer – heart disease.

He has been featured on radio programs and online shows; he has also been featured or quoted in print publications. For more information on this author, including his workout DVD, "Take Exercise to Heart," go to Joe's website (www.exercisetoheart.com).

CPSIA information can be obtained at www.ICGtesting.com
Printed in the USA
BVOW01s1103160814

362841BV00008B/17/P